SHUFFLEBOARD
WHY NOT?

BY

JOHN MATAYA

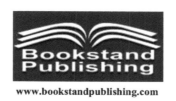

www.bookstandpublishing.com

Published by
Bookstand Publishing
Morgan Hill, CA 95037
3328_15

ISBN 978-1-58909-908-1

Printed in the United States of America

Acknowledgements

I, gratefully acknowledge the contributions of a great number of officers, directors from the local and county levels, State of Florida and National Associations who have spent numerous hours for the benefit of Shuffleboard.

Also, I want to thank the many un-recognized workers, who maintain the courts, discs and other equipment required to make this game a pleasure to play.

I am grateful to the many opponents who have helped me to become a better player, correct my faults, separate the good from the bad and to recognize that Shuffleboard is 85% mental and 15% physical.

Thanks to the authors of the following Shuffleboard Books for their knowledge and instructions on how to play Shuffleboard;

- "How to Book of Shuffleboard," by Charles S. Haslam, Copyright 1977, by Great Outdoors Publishing Co.
- "Secrets of Shuffleboard Strategy," by Omero C. Catan, Second Edition, Copyright 1967, 1968 and 1973 by Omero C. Catan.
- "Shuffleboard, Those Capricious Discs," by Floyd W. Swem, Copyright 1980, by Great Outdoors Publishing Co.
- "Modular Shuffleboard," by Wilbur L. Estes, Copyright 1995, by Wilbur L. Estes.

Special thanks to Charles Crescimanno, Ray Russmann, Richard Rosen, Antonio Manzo, Vernon Uzzell, Vito Chieco and to all the other excellent Shuffleboard players who love the game.

Many, many thanks to Jeanette Lundy for her love, friendship, companionship and her untiring effort to help produce this book.

Shuffleboard, **WHY NOT** ?? Is dedicated to:

My deceased parents:	Lawrence and Pauline Mataya
My deceased wife:	Grace Mataya
My children:	Perry Mataya, wife Xinli, children John, Eleanor, Olivia
	Wendy Mataya, daughter, Virginia Grace
My significant other:	Jeanette Lundy, her daughter, Denise Purcell, husband Rick, son Ryan

ABOUT the AUTHOR:

John L. Mataya has been involved with Shuffleboard since 1997, as a player, team captain, teaching beginners how to play, in an administrative capacity and club president of the Shuffleboard Club, located in the retirement community of On-Top-of-The World, Ocala, Florida. He has a reputation for practical advice, technical accuracy, as well as the ability to explain a variety of complex topics.

He started to play shuffleboard in 1997, age 70, in the retirement community of Oak Run, Ocala, Florida. Played annually in Marion County, Ocala Senior Center Games, 1998 to 2003. State of Florida Senior Games: The Villages, 2004 / Leesburg, 2005 / Cape Coral, 2006, 2007, 2008, 2009. Qualified for the National Senior Games, Louisville, Kentucky 2007, withdrew because of illness. Played in the National Senior Games, Stanford University, Palo Alto, California, 2009, 4th in Singles, 1st in Doubles, age 82.

In his younger years, played high school football/basketball/softball/tennis and croquet. US Army, Corps of Engineers, honorable discharged October 1946. Graduated from University of Illinois, Urbana, IL. B.S. Civil Engineer, June 1951. State of Illinois: Registered Structural Engineer, Professional Engineer and Registered Architect all by examination. Worked as an Architect and Engineer with some of the largest Arch/Eng firms in Chicago, IL. With the A/E firm Skidmore Owings and Merrill, on the design team, Air Force Academy, Colorado Springs, Colorado.

He married Grace Weigold, April 1961, started his own Architect/Engineer Firm, June 1962, 2-children, boy/girl, started his 2nd childhood, learned to cross-country ski/ice skate/golf/bowl and camping.

March 1983, began working for the US Government, General Service Administration, retired as Contracting Officer, GS-14 for Architectural/Engineering contracts in the National Capital Region, Washington, D.C. Sept. 1994.

With the children gone, John and Grace moved to Florida to the retirement community of Oak Run in 1997. In January 1998, his wife of 36 years suddenly dies, leaving him to begin a new life.

Starting a new life playing cards/golf/bocce ball and shuffleboard during which time he met Jeanette Lundy, a widow of 6 years, who also played bocce ball and shuffleboard. From friendship to romance and the start of a new life.

His 3rd childhood, play and more play, 24/7 in a new retirement community, On Top-of-The World with new furniture, new friends and activities.

Shuffleboard, always a fun game, requires judgment and discipline to win. See you on the Shuffleboard court.

CONTENTS

Contents

Contents

INTRODUCTION

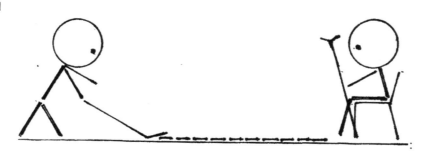

   SHUFFLEBOARD!!! *"WHY Not"*??? It's a sport for active people. It's similar to a game we all played as a child, called "hide-and-go-seek," plus playing on a surface to score points to win.
   Shuffleboard is not your typical game like Basketball/Football/Tennis/Golf/Baseball or Softball. Why? Because, you can start to learn the game at age 55. The 2009 Summer National Senior Games at Stanford University, Palo Alto, CA, August 1-15, had 153 Shuffleboard players, aged from 50-90 from 20 states.
   At 55, people retire and ask themselves, *"What do I do next?"* Play Shuffleboard! Are you kidding me! Not my game, time out!

   The majority of competitive sports, basketball/football/golf/baseball/tennis starts at an early age and continues to around the age of 45 to 50. Your physical body is not able to keep up with the young players in their prime. Shuffleboard is a sport which embraces both the mind and body. Yes, your *"mind"* is sharp and the desire is there, but not the physical body. You need to *reconsider*; *regroup* and change *directions*. Starting at age 55, Shuffleboard can do this for you.

   Things to consider:

A. The Start/End of player's competitive career in most competitive sports is from age 15 – 45.
B. The PEAK of one's physical competitive career in all competitive sports is: Age 30.+/-

C. The span of reflection/review/change of direction/mental/physical health is from age 45 – 60.

D. Shuffleboard, the Start/End to make the use of one's mental/physical health is from age 60 – 90.
E. The PEAK of a player's mental/physical ability is: Age 75.+/-

   Graph of typical person's competitive sports activity is as follows:

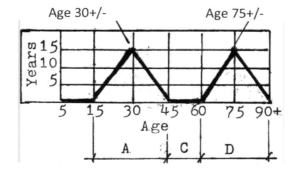

INTRODUCTION

Shuffleboard History:

In 1913, modern shuffleboard came to Daytona Beach, Florida. The courts were packed sand with wood disc, 5 ½ inches diameter and 7/8 inch thick. The cues were wood with a notched block with a wood handle on a 6 foot stick. To increase control of the wooden discs, the packed sand was replaced with a concrete surface.

In 1922, W.N. Britton from Daytona Beach, came to St. Petersburg, Florida and suggested the city officials build a shuffleboard court and use the game as a tourist attraction. In 1923, P.T. Ives of St. Petersburg, built a shuffleboard court and in January 24, 1924 the Mirror Lake Shuffleboard Club was organized. The next four years over 1,300 members of the club played on 28 concrete courts.

December 12, 1928, E.F. Wolfrum, President of the Mirror Lake Shuffleboard Club, met with 10 members of the club in St. Petersburg to form the *Florida Shuffleboard Association* to establish uniform rules for the game. The Florida State organization paved the way for the organization of the *National Shuffleboard Association*. February 24, 1931, the first National Shuffleboard Association was formed with E.F. Wolfrum as president. The first official act was to announce the President's Cup to be played annually, summer and winter. C.L. Bailey was the first winner of the President's Cup in the first tournament held in St. Petersburg, March 1931.

1959. The National Shuffleboard Hall of Fame, was located at Mirror Lake Shuffleboard Club, St. Petersburg, Florida. 1972, a permanent building was erected to house the exhibit at the Mirror Lake Park Shuffleboard Club.

Currently, the Mirror Lake Park exhibit has been re-located to Clearwater, Florida and is now called the *International and National Hall of Fame.* Located at the *Lawn Bowls and Shuffleboard Complex.* 1020 Calumet St., Clearwater, Florida 33755. Phone: 727 446-3306, www. Clearwater-fl.com. Visitors can take a self-guided walk through the history of the sport/awards/pictures/articles and equipment. Guided tours upon request.

Shuffleboard, WHY NOT ? is written for the beginning player, who wants to improve his/her shuffleboard game to the best of their individual abilities. The information herein, has many illustrations which are presented with humor/clarity and sufficient detail to hold the beginners or advanced player's interest in becoming the "player" you originally thought you were.

Every Shuffleboard player can shoot as well as the next, the difference in the player is the margin of strategic knowledge one has learned to retain and use. Shuffleboard is 85% strategy and 15% skill. Shuffleboard is a sport you have to participate in before you can intelligently say, it's *good* or *bad*. Have fun, play *Shuffleboard*, WHY NOT?

PLAYER REQUIREMENTS :

1. Playing Court:

The Court/Tools/Clothing as required for 2, 3 or 4 persons to play the game of shuffleboard is as follows:

     1.   Playing Court
     2.   Set of 8-Waxed Discs/Cue Sticks
     3.   Score Board/Chalk/Eraser
     4.   Scoring
     5.   Clothing/Shoes

Shuffleboard is generally played outdoors on a concrete slab which has a playing area 6 feet wide and 39 feet long. A standing area for the players to shoot from 6 feet-6 inches at each end plus a 2" higher raised slab 4 feet to stop the discs from going off the playing court and used for player seating. When two or more courts are constructed the court will be separated by a 2' alley which slopes from zero at the <u>Head</u> or <u>Foot</u> towards the middle to a storm water drain. See FIGURES 1, 2 and 3.

     The court is marked with a <u>HEAD</u> and a <u>FOOT</u>. With the score board located at the HEAD end and on the <u>YELLOW</u> player side.

Any Disc that is in the DEAD zone (12' at mid-court) is removed from the court. If it touches the line in the direction of play it remains.

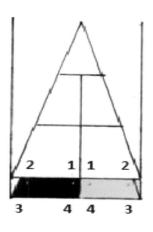 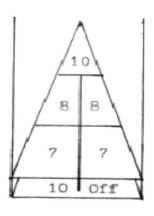

Shooting Position	Scoring Area
FIGURE 2	FIGURE 3

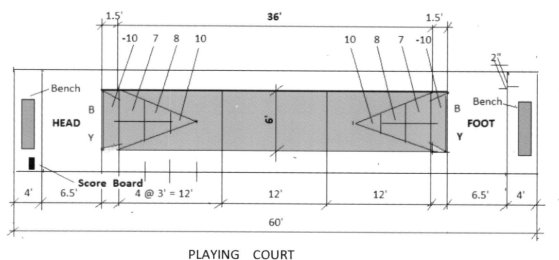

PLAYING COURT
FIGURE 1

PLAYER REQUIREMENTS:

2. DISCS/CUE STICKS:

Discs: Set of discs in accordance with the National Shuffleboard Association shall be made of molded phenolic composition not less than 1 inch in thickness, 6 inches in diameter, and not less than 11½ ounces in weight. New discs shall weigh 15 ounces. Four (4) discs shall be colored **YELLOW**, four (4) **BLACK**. These eight discs comprise a set. See Figure 4.

Discs are waxed with a disc wax stick which aids the disc in sliding on the concrete surface. Manually the wax stick is used by rubbing the bottom of the disc six (6) times horizontal and six (6) vertical lines across each disc before play. The same procedure is used for waxing the discs using an electric brush polisher. Beads made of silicon may also be used to aid the disc to slide on the concrete surface. Each shuffleboard club uses some type of wax or beads to improve play.

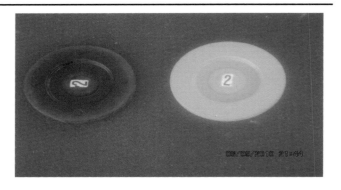

FIGURE 4

reduces friction, noise and better shots. The shafts are aluminum or fiberglass, the fiberglass shaft is lighter and recommended. On one end of the cue shaft is the handle with a rubber tip, used to move and arrange the discs after the play at the Head or Foot has finished. The **H**ead of the cue used for shooting the disc should **not** be used to move or arrange discs, this could damage the alignment of the Cue Head. See Figure 5 and 6.

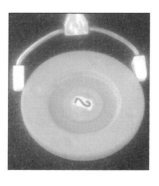

Cue Stick NIBS in contact with
Shuffleboard 6" diameter disc

FIGURE 5

Cue Sick: The national rules require the cue to be no more than six feet, 3 inches (6'-3"). No metal part of the cue shall touch the playing surface of the court. Cues are of two basic types: the rider or the glider. The rider has a cross-piece which sits on top of the disc with delrin buttons. It rides the disc and does not touch the court. The glider cue has a steel head with delrin keystone runners. The delrin runners swivel, lying flat through the shuffling stroke which

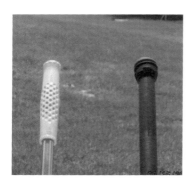

Typical Handles

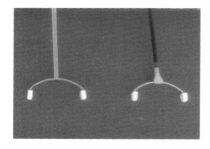

Typical CUE STICKS

FIGURE 6

PLAYER REQUIREMENTS:

3. *Score Board/Chalk/Eraser*:

Score Board; The National Shuffleboard Association adopted the universal scoreboard, designed by George Merz. The unique feature of the scoreboard, the four (4) color selector, which shows what is being played. They are:

Position 1. Doubles, first game, YELLOW out first at each end of the court.
Position 2. Doubles, second game, BLACK out first at each end of the court.
Position 3. Walking, singles, first game, YELLOW out first at the Head of the court; BLACK out at the Foot.
Position 4. Walking, singles, second game. BLACK out first at the Head of the court; YELLOW out at the Foot.

Non-walking singles game, the players at the Head of the court use the two (2) left-hand columns to record their scores: the players at the Foot of the court use the two (2) right-hand columns to record their scores.

The information from the Score Board is as Follows;
1. The score of each player at the moment.
2. The player which has the first shot in the frame being played.
3. The number of frames being played. (If a point game, the number of frames is not important).

The success of many games depends on the selection of the correct shot to be made. Therefore: the beginner, casual or intermediate players, need to **LOOK at the SCORE BOARD before they SHOOT!**

Chalk/Eraser:

Chalk/Eraser: is used to change the score on the score board and the eraser to correct the mistakes. Often players need help to add/subtract, because you could have a minus 10, 3 or 2. If you have a minus

score, high-light it with a circle drawn around the score so it can be seen by both the Head/Foot players.

4. *Scoring/Hand Signals:*

Scoring: The person shooting the YELLOW disc is the score keeper. The YELLOW **score** is always read first and the BLACK score last. For example; the score for first frame, YELLOW Head 7, BLACK 8. First frame, Foot score YELLOW 7, BLACK minus 10. The new score in frame # 2; YELLOW 14 (7+7) and BLACK is minus 2 (-2), (-10 +8=-2). A circle is drawn around the minus 2 to clearly identify BLACK is in the hole by 2-points.

Example: score board design, plus above scores. See Figure 7.

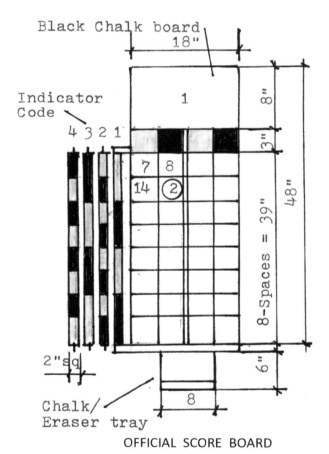

OFFICIAL SCORE BOARD

FIGURE 7

PLAYER REQUIREMENTS :

Hand Signals:

Hand Signals: The hand signal for *no-score*, move the right hand with the fingers together and bring the arm, waist high, across the waist back and forth several times.

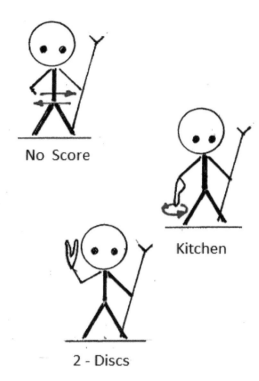

No Score

The signal for a disc in the *Kitchen* (minus 10). Drop the right arm down with the index finger pointing towards the ground and rotate the arm in a circle several times.

Kitchen

To tell the opposite end of the playing court, Head/Foot, which discs are good in the scoring area. Hold up the right arm with the fingers closed, open up 1, 2 or 3 fingers in the up position to indicate the number of good discs. The color of the discs is not important because the players can see which colors are good. Hand signals are used to keep from shouting the position of the discs which can be disturbing to players on adjacent courts.

2 - Discs

Clothing/Shoes:

Clothing:

Clothing: should be casual, comfortable and suitable for the climate. Sun glasses and a cap with a visor in bright sun light.

Shoes:

Shoes: should be tennis shoes, walking shoes, but not street shoes with a hard sole, or flip- flops with open toes. Hard sole shoes can scar the court playing surface and open-toes can be hit by flying discs.

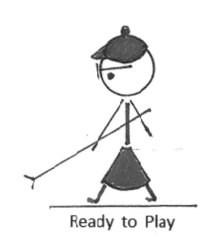

Ready to Play

BASIC KNOWLEDGE :

Number of DISCS in the SCORING AREA:

BASIC Knowledge; To determine how many discs each scoring area, 10/8/7 will hold to count for score without touching a line. Beginners and many players say the 10 area will hold 2 or up to 4 discs.

Theoretically the 10/8/7-area will hold the following number of discs;

The **10-area** will hold **8-discs**. In actual play, 3 or 2, mostly 1; because the opponent will knock the disc out and try to stick their disc for a 10.

The **8-area** will hold **14 discs**. The **7-area** will hold **26 discs**. In actual play the most in one frame would be 8 discs, 4-YELLOW and 4-BLACK. See Figure 8.

The lesson: If you have the last shot and you want to score, the 8 or 7-area gives you a better chance of scoring, than trying to score a 10. Discipline and judgment is a better route to follow to win.

The 10-area becomes important as the game gets closer to 75 or the last frame, as a hammer or as bait.
The 7- area can hold more discs than the 10 or the 8-area. Also, the 7-area has <u>56%</u> more area than the 10 or 8 area. See Figure 9.

How can the theoretical scoring of discs be of use to a player?
(A) Increase the player's confidence.
(B) Better and quicker shot selection, knowing the odds of success.

In actual play, the player with the hammer, on the last shot, has to decide which area they want to shoot a disc into for score.

1. The <u>8-area is 3 times greater</u> than the <u>10-area</u>, the <u>7-area is 5 times greater</u> than the <u>10-area</u>. The <u>7-area is 2 times greater</u> than the <u>8-area</u>. See Figure 9.

The use of the 8 or 7-area will produce greater results than the use of the 10-area.

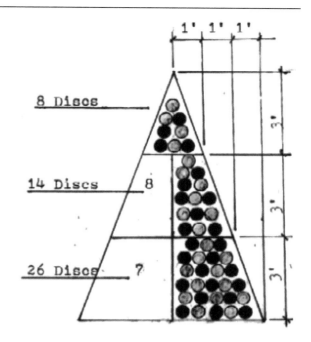

NUMBER of GOOD DISCS in the SCORING AREA

FIGURE 8

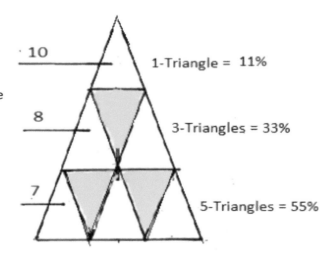

% CHANGE of SCORING in the 10/8/7 AREA

FIGURE 9

BASIC KNOWLEDGE:

TASTE of STROKE with CUE STICK:

Shuffleboard, like golf, for the beginning player, starts at the driving range, to get the mechanics of hitting a golf ball on the driving range. Shuffleboard, for the beginning player, starts by trying to use the correct grip, (right hand-right foot), to push the disc into the 7/8 or 10 scoring area and to get the feel of shuffling.

The play begins at the Head by placing 4-YELLOW discs and 4-BLACK discs into the hitting area.

One player at the Head and the second player goes to the Foot of the playing court to remove the discs away from the 7-scoring area. The drill: shoot one YELLOW disc at a time into the 7-scoring area. Like shooting free-throws in basketball. The player shoots all 4-YELLOW discs, 4 is perfect. Next, the player shoots the 4-BLACK discs, one at a time into the 8-scoring area, 4 being perfect.

The person at the Foot, places the YELLOW/ BLACK discs into the shooting box and shoots one disc at a time towards the YELLOW 7 and the BLACK 8-scoring area, with 4 discs in each area being perfect.

The person at the YELLOW Head puts 4-discs in the shooting area and tries to place one disc at a time into the 10-scoring area for a perfect score of 4. The player at the Foot will return the 4-YELLOW disc into the 10-scoring area for perfect score of 4. The total score for the game is 12. See Figure 10 for an example.

This beginning introduction into shooting for distance and scoring is good practice and a confidence builder for beginners and intermediate players. This drill should take place before playing a real game.

At one of our "Introduction to Shuffleboard Sessions," for new players, we had a two (2) shots get one (1) disc into the 7-scoring area and win a 1-year free-pass to league play. In a 4-hour period, we had zero winners. Why? Shuffleboard, like golf, the beginner needs instructions on how to hold the cue stick, the stroke, guidance on how to play and the importance of practice.

Later in the game of 40, 10 different shots are used to aid all players to become better through practice.

Example; beginners shooting discs into the 7, 8 and 10 scoring area and keeping score. See Figure 10.

SCORE BOARD

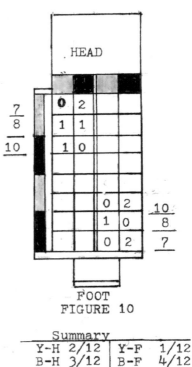

FOOT
FIGURE 10

Summary			
Y-H 2/12	Y-F 1/12
B-H 3/12	B-F 4/12

BASIC KNOWLEDGE :

HEAD/FOOT: Where to GO.

Shuffleboard: doubles (4-players) two (2) at the Head and two (2) at the Foot. With only three (3) players the game is the same, except the third player is the walker and plays both Head and Foot. Singles (match play) is similar to doubles play except each player shoots the YELLOW or BLACK discs at the Head or Foot.

The shuffleboard game is started by the player shooting the YELLOW disc at the Head of the playing court. Also, they are the score keeper. In league play, chips or cards are drawn to see which player is the YELLOW Head, the BLACK Head, the YELLOW Foot and the BLACK Foot. Generally you play three (3) games with a score of 75 or 16 frames. If a score of 75 is first the game is over. In tournament play, see rule C-2c for YELLOW or BLACK.

The chart plan for player position for each game is generally posted near the Head/Foot of the court.

If the YELLOW Head player stays at the YELLOW Head for **three** (3) games, each player plays one (1) time with the YELLOW Head player. The player positions are as follows; See **Example # 1.**

Player	GAME #1	GAME #2	GAME #3
1	Y-Head	Y-Head	Y-Head
2	B-Head	Y-Foot	B-Foot
3	B-Foot	B-head	Y-Foot
4	Y-Foot	B-Foot	B-Head

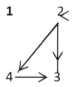

Each player, 2, 3 & 4 play one time with the **# 1** player. They rotate counter-clock-wise.

If the YELLOW player stays at YELLOW Head for two (2) games, each player plays one (1) time with each player. The positions are as follows: See **Example # 2**.

	GAME #1	GAME #2	GAME #3
1	Y-Head	Y-Head	B-Foot
2	B-Head	Y-Foot	Y-Head
3	Y-Foot	B-Foot	Y-Foot
4	B-Foot	B-Head	B-Head

```
     1      2   |  1      4   |  2      4
                |      ↙ ↓    |   ↓    ↘
     3      4   |  2  →  3    |  3  ←  1

Game #  1          2              3
```

Each player, 2, 3 & 4 play one time with the **# 1** player.

The score for three (3) games with 4-players is as follows;

If one player wins three (3) games the score for each player is **3+1+1+1= 6, total for 3- games**.

If one player wins two (2) games the score for each player is **2+2+2+0= 6, total for 3-games.**

The score for three (3) games with 3-players.

One (1) player walks each game, the score is as follows;

If each walker wins, the score for each player is **2+2+2= 6, total for 3-games in lieu of 1+1+1= 3.**

If two (2) walkers win and one (1) walker does not the score for each player is **3+3+0= 6, total for 3-games.**

If one (1) walker wins and two (2) walkers do not win, the score for each player is **4+1+1= 6, total for 3-games.**

If three (3) walkers loose, the score for each player is **2+2+2= 6, total for 3-games.**

BASIC KNOWLEDGE :

BEGINNING GAME: St Pete/Tampa

Shuffleboard, a game of "Hide-an-seek" starts with the person shooting YELLOW. The YELLOW player looks at the playing court and says to themselves! **Where do I Hide?** The playing court is blank, no hiding place. Hence; a hiding place must be created. Otherwise, BLACK will knock my YELLOW disc off the playing area, also you need to score points to win.

Good ole **St. Pete** (Cross-Block), YELLOW player going to place a disc on the St. Pete position on BLACK's side of the playing court, to hide YELLOW's second shot behind the St. Pete block. Good thinking!!!

The correct placement of the first YELLOW disc to start the hide is half-way between the apex of the playing triangle and the playing edge of the court. The distance from the point of the triangle to the outer edge is 3 feet, to the middle is 1½ feet. To place the YELLOW disc in this position takes a lot of practice. How important is this shot? This is the # 4 shot in ones' shot vocabulary. Every player has to be able to <u>execute</u> this shot to win. See Figure 11.

BLACK's turn to shoot. The options that the BLACK player has are as follows:

Option #1; BLACK can shoot the first disc down the outer edge of the playing court to count for a score in the 7-scoring area. This shot is known as down "suicide alley," Why? It's a very difficult shot to score in the 7-scoring area. On a score of 1 to 5, it rates a 2. See Figure 11.

Option #2; BLACK elects to hit the YELLOW disc and put the disc into the kitchen, or hit the disc with a carom shot and remove the disc from the playing area, with their disc going off the board. On a score of 1 to 5, it rates a 2. Why? To put the YELLOW disc into the kitchen it's more luck than skill. They could stick and leave the YELLOW disc in the 7-scoring area, which would be bad luck. A carom hit of the YELLOW disc could knock the disc off the court, but their disc may glance off to the YELLOW side of the court to give YELLOW a hide. See Figure 11.

Option #3; BLACK can put a BLACK disc on the right side of the YELLOW disc which will "block," YELLOW's next shot for hide behind their YELLOW disc. On a scale of 1 to 5, it rates as 5. Why? Now YELLOW has to make another choice as to where to shoot to. See Figure 11.

Option #4; BLACK, with a carom shot can knock off the YELLOW disc and their disc also, BLACK has the hammer, which would make YELLOW set up another St. Pete. On a scale of 1 to 5, it rates a 3. Why? Carom shots take a lot of practice. The better strategy is to block and let YELLOW decide what to do, who knows, he may set up a pigeon shot for you. The Head YELLOW/BLACK part of the "<u>opening shots</u>" is completed and now the YELLOW/BLACK Foot players have to play their opening game.

Physiology is an important part of the game and each player must make it work for you. Nothing goes wrong, because a "mistake" isn't damaging, unless it is repeated. Shuffleboard is a game of percentages and not of perfection.

Discipline, in shuffleboard will help the player try to do "<u>only</u>" what needs to be done. A mistake is caused by the lack of knowledge, or the lack of experience and discipline. It is important to play against better players. However, if the better player doesn't play their best, the beginner learns nothing of value.

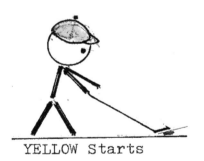
YELLOW Starts

BASIC KNOWLEDGE:

BEGINNING GAME: St Pete/Tampa

The next choice the YELLOW player has to start the game is the Tampa shot. The Tampa is placed on the player's side of the playing court at the apex of the triangle. See Figure 12 for the exact location. The importance of this shot in a player's vocabulary is number-5. A great deal of practice is required to get the shot in the correct position. A slight miss-placement often results in a hide for your opponent.

If the YELLOW shot is placed correctly, the next YELLOW shot would be "deep" into the 7-scoring area and as near to the vertical line between the 7-scoring area without touching the vertical line for a hide.

Black shoots next; They have only "**one**" shot. They must **"clear"** the Tampa off the scoring area and make the YELLOW player set-up again! The opening game has ended and the middle game begins.

Once the Tampa is cleared, YELLOW may set-up again. If YELLOW sets-up again. BLACK, again clears the Tampa off the scoring area.

YELLOW's third disc may be shot into the 7-scoring area on YELLOW's side, as deep and near to the outside corner of the 7-scoring area as possible. BLACK has to shoot a very long cross-court shot to clear the YELLOW disc. If BLACK's shot is off, it may carom off and slide into the kitchen.

If BLACK's third shot clears the board, YELLOW's fourth shot is into the 10-scoring area as near to the apex as possible, forcing BLACK to clear the YELLOW for a no-score frame.

As a general rule, do not use a Tampa when you are ahead. If you are behind, place a Tampa with the third disc, your opponent may clear and stick. If the score is 65 or more, try a Tampa with your first disc, the opponent may stick. Remember, every play that works for you, also works for your opponent. All shuffleboard players make "dumb" mistakes. A mistake doesn't hurt unless it is repeated. Use your mistakes to gain experience and confidence.

The Middle Game:

The strategy in the middle game is score if the opponent scores. Keep the score as close as possible.

Why? If the yellow is down 20 points, this can be made up in one (1) round. Example; YELLOW scores a 7 and 8 for a 15, BLACK scores a zero, YELLOW is down only 5 points. If the YELLOW is down 30 points, it takes two (2) rounds to catch up. Example; YELLOW scores a 10 and 7 for 17, BLACK scores a zero, YELLOW is down 13 points.

Yellow no longer has the option of scoring. The opponent's score has to be reduced to keep the game alive and out of reach. Thus, the secret weapon, the "kitchen shot," to put BLACK into the kitchen for a minus 10. Example; BLACK a minus 10, YELLOW a 7 + 8 = 15, the score 15 to 30, YELLOW down 15 points, it takes 3-rounds to catch up.

From physics, a body at "rest" tends to remain at rest and for every action there is an equal and opposite reaction. The kitchen shot must hit the disc at rest with enough energy to move the disc into the minus 10 area and remain at the point of contact for a score or carom off the court. If the opponent's disc is in the 7 scoring area, the disc is hit with enough speed to move the sitting disc 2 to 2 ½ feet. Practice to get the "feel" of this shot. Also, shooting the disc in the 8 or 10 scoring area takes more speed and accuracy than to put the opponent's disc into the minus 10 area.

In the middle game, keep the "table clean." If you can see the opponent's disc, shoot at it! Try to knock their disc off the playing area or catch a line for no score. The **hammer** is the number one (1) disc and the **kitchen shot** the number two (2) disc of the middle game. If YELLOW should shoot their disc for a "perfect," minus 10, they should refrain from trying to knock out the minus 10 with a second disc because they may stick. Place a disc in the 8 or 7, for a loss of 2 or 3 points in lieu of a 10.

BASIC KNOWLEDGE:

BEGINNING GAME: St. Pete/Tampa Placement

The disc into the 10-area is the number <u>three (3)</u> <u>shot</u>, because it can be used for a score or a hide. Remember, the 10-area can hold 8 discs. Look for the opponent's backstop/horizontal double on the 10/8 line.

Tampa is an alternate shot for the St. Pete. Why? YELLOW disc # 1 and 3 are shot as St. Pete's.

BLACK cleared disc # 1 and # 3. YELLOW shot disc # 5 for a Tampa. BLACK may try to clear, but sticks, which gives YELLOW disc # 7 a hide. See Figure 11 for a St. Pete and Figure 12 for a Tampa hide.

St. PETE

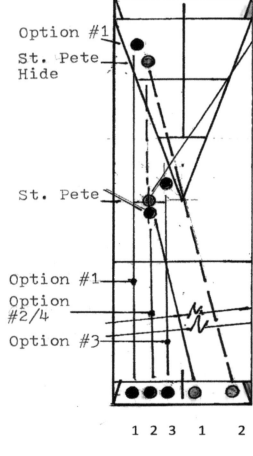

HEAD
FIGURE 11

TAMPA

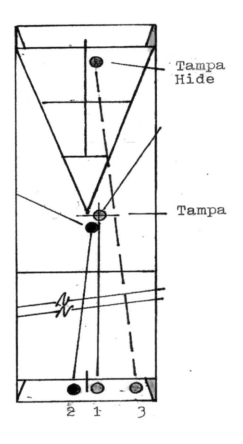

HEAD
FIGURE 12

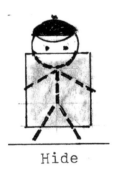

Hide

12

GRIP / STROKE:

Grip/ Stroke:

Grip:

The shuffleboard grip is similar to the golf grip. The whole body, plus the correct grip, is required to play consistent and uniform shuffleboard.

The grip for a right hand player is as follows:

Place three (3) fingers around the cue stick with the thumb directly on top of the cue stick and the little finger at the very end of the grip. The player stands erect and relaxed, with both feet parallel to the minus 10 line with the right arm straight down their right side. The cue "*nibs*" must be around the disc to be shot. The amount of pressure exerted by the right hand on the cue stick is very little. The cue stick could fall out of the player's grip, it is that loose. The player's eyes leave the cue stick and become *fixed* on the target until the disc leaves the cue stick. See Figure 13.

For a left side player, the same directions only on the opposite side.

1. Poor aiming technique, lack of focus on target.
2. Throwing out the shooting arm
3. The follow through
4. The fast shot, to remove a kitchen disc
5. Taking a "peek" at disc before shooting
6. Changing your mind
7. Tension, loss of composure
8. Distraction, external etc.

To play better, you need to be constantly aware of the list of problems associated with the shooting of the disc. Some of the common distractions are:

1. Shooting past your opponent's block to clear their good score.
2. Shooting for a score when the opponent's disc is near yours on a line.
3. Shooting the hammer, last shot, to win!

As a beginning player, the more games played, tension/distractions/ concentration is a basic part of the shuffleboard game. Experience and practice will help, "do what you need to do to win".

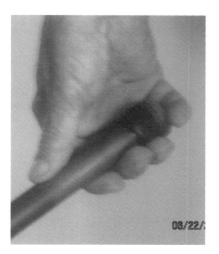

FIGURE 13

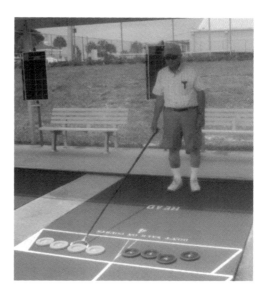

Ready to SHOOT !

All of the published Shuffleboard books write about the common problems of delivery. They are as follows:

GRIP / STROKE:

Stroke:

The delivery: Every shuffleboard player needs to learn how to use a cue stick. The beginner needs to learn about direction/ distance/ speed to reach the intended target. <u>How to do this?</u> Players take many shapes and styles. The grip/ body /arm movement are similar and alike for all that play shuffleboard. The correct delivery for every player can not be presented.

Stroke: The player looks at the target, takes a step and another step, the body bent forward towards the intended target. Moves the cue stick from the shoulder of the Right arm, towards the target. The speed of the delivery is controlled by the Right arm. The Left-handed player is the same, but the opposite side.

The mechanics of the "**Stance/Stroke and Follow Through**" for the *Right arm-Left foot* follow through versus the *Right arm-Right foot* follow through are as shown. See Figure 14. (A) and (B).

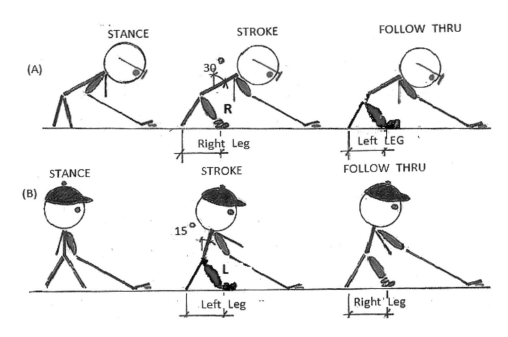

FIGURE 14

(A). The stance/stroke and follow through, <u>Right arm-Left leg</u> often used by many players.

(B). The stance/stroke and follow through, <u>Right arm-Right Leg</u> is **preferred** because:

1. The <u>Right arm-Right Leg body</u> and arm movement is more erect and the delivery is on the same plane.
2. <u>Right arm-Right Leg</u> helps to keep the Right arm from flying.
3. The head is more erect and easier to concentrate and focus on the target.
4.   A tendency to rotate the body when the <u>Right arm-Left foot,</u> is used to increase speed to a target.
5. <u>Right arm-Left leg</u> the delivery is made with two (2) body planes, in lieu of one (1) for Right arm-Right Leg.

Keep the stroke **SIMPLE** and increase the accuracy!

KITCHEN PLAY:

Kitchen – Good/Bad!

Kitchen play is a major part of the Shuffleboard game. Why? To place your opponent's disc into the kitchen will reduce the score and change the game.

The kitchen depth is <u>1'-6"</u> where the depth of the 8/7 area is <u>3'.</u> The accuracy required to place a disc into the 10-off area is <u>twice</u> as difficult as trying to score an 8 or 7.

Beginners love to kitchen: they want to master the game, which becomes a primary goal. **Rule:** play kitchen only when you are <u>behind</u> and <u>need</u> to reduce your opponent's score

When to play Kitchen Bait? When you are behind, 14-20 points (2 frames) to catch up, or sooner, if near the end of the game. If 10 points behind, the kitchen shot is not required. Use disc #6 to bait. If your opponent fails to clear, or puts you in the kitchen and their disc sticks for a score, use your last disc to reverse the score.

The opponent misses the Kitchen bait, yes it <u>does happen</u>, you should not place a guard for the bait. Instead place another disc in the opposite 7-area, far away, to discourage a combination shot.

If the opponent's kitchens one (1) of the baits and sticks. You should ignore the unprotected 7 bait and put the opponent's disc into the kitchen. If the opponent's disc doesn't stick and clears one of the 7 baits, score another 7, if your last disc, score an 8.

If the opponent shoots their disc into the kitchen. What should you do? In a <u>frame game</u>, block the 10-Off disc with a disc in the no scoring area of the board. Also consider the condition of the court and how deep the disc is in the kitchen. If the court is slow and the disc is deep go for score far away from the 10-Off and let the opponent decide what to do.

Where to place the Kitchen Bait?

The Kitchen bait is placed in the low 7-area

for the following reasons:

1. Deep in the 7-area, hard for the opponent to clear the disc off the board, plus they may stick.

2. The opponent decides to put your disc into the Kitchen, their disc stops close to the 7-area for a score. You can bump their disc into the kitchen and knock your disc out and score.

3. With the bait in the low 7-area, there is a good chance of the opponent placing their own disc into the kitchen. See Figure 15.

4. Place the St. Pete, then place the kitchen bait on the opposite side of the St. Pete. Why? To prevent the opponent's disc from being protected by your St. Pete. See Figure 16.

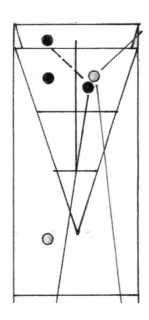
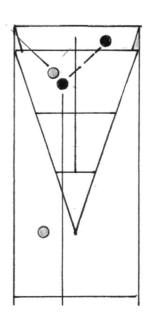

FIGURE 16   FIGURE 15

15

KITCHEN PLAY:

Kitchen Play: Some things to consider about Kitchen Play!

1.   Your opponent is <u>ahead</u> and in the <u>kitchen</u>, place your third disc (3) deep into the <u>10-area</u>, they may clear the 10 and stick, use their disc as a backstop and score your disc for a 10. Read the Score Board <u>first</u>.

2.   Place a <u>low 8</u> on the opponent side, they can clear and roll for a hide behind your St. Pete. Use your disc to put them into the kitchen. Good strategy when the opponent clears everything.

3.   <u>Sucker's Hide:</u> to <u>lure</u> the opponent onto the board, you offer it when they are ahead and you need a kitchen to keep the game alive. The <u>prime purpose</u>, get the opponent on the board when they <u>do not</u> need to. If they do, the strategy is a success.

4.   <u>Gift of a 7:</u> Try to put your opponent's St. Pete or Tampa into the kitchen and <u>fall short</u>, leaving the target disc in the 7-area for a score. Now they have two (2) discs on the board, the original hide behind the St. Pete and the friendly 7. Try a combination shot to clear the board and put the other one into the kitchen or a direct kitchen shot for one disc. See Figure 17.

5.   <u>Reverse the order of play:</u> You have the the hammer, place your opponent's St. Pete into the kitchen. They knock the kitchened disc out, but you set up your own St.Pete, reversing the order of play. A difficult shot to make.

6.   <u>Short St. Pete:</u> The opponent has the hammer, your shot is short of the Lag line, trying to set a high St. Pete. Your disc is removed, You are surprised, you failed, the opponent sets a good St. Pete or Tampa. You now have a chance to put a good 7 behind their St.Pete for a score.

7.   <u>Intentional Stick:</u> You have the hammer, the opponent sets a St. Pete or Tampa. You try to clear and stick, <u>creating a Sucker's hide</u>. Your opponent tries to hide behind the new St. Pete, you can now clear and score.

8.   <u>Suicide Alley</u>; when behind, place kitchen bait near the 8/7 line, but do not go into the 7-area. They may try to clear and leave their disc in the 7-area. This sets up a combination shot by bumping your suicide disc into their 7 for a kitchen and a score.

To improve your Game:

Rule No. 1: When you are <u>ahead</u> and your score is **43,** do not hide (sneak). Why? Your opponent is losing. They need to keep the game going with a Kitchen. Use score of 43 as a guide for control and proper conduct of your game.

Rule No. 2: Do not place Kitchen Bait when your opponent <u>has the hammer</u> and the score is between <u>50 and 60</u>. Why? Desire, <u>not need</u>, controls the play of most players. Hence, play as if your opponent will try to end the game.

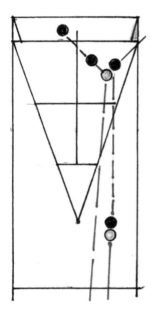

FIGURE 17

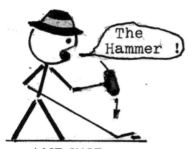

LAST SHOT

GUARDS/HIDES :

Guards/Blocks:

Guards: Protective, a St. Pete or a Tampa, used to protect the next shot of the player. **Blocks:** used to prevent the anticipated shot by the opponent.

The Tampa used after the St. Pete has been cleared from the board twice. Use your third disc to set a Tampa. Before the opponent clears the Tampa they should consider the following :

1. Do not bump the Tampa into the 7-area for a score.
2. Do not stick cue disc and leave a block.
3. Do not let either disc glance to a place for a good hide for the other player. See FIGURE 18 and FIGURE 19.

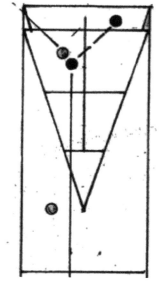

FIGURE 19

BLACK places a St. Pete off to the right of the correct position. YELLOW puts up a Tampa at the 10-area apex. BLACK's hide stops at the 8/7 line which is blocked by the Tampa. If the Tampa is knocked away, BLACK could score a double. Also this condition could result if the hide was on the 10/8 line. See Figure 19.

FIGURE   18

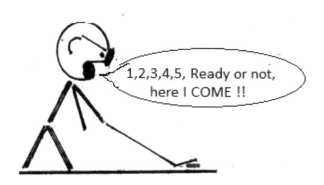

1,2,3,4,5, Ready or not, here I COME !!

GUARDS/HIDES:

The Tampa can be used to fill in: place the Tampa on the opponent's side of the BLACK'S St. Pete to prevent BLACK from placing a disc for a hide. See FIGURE 20.

BLACK places a St. Pete too deep. YELLOW puts a Tampa at the 10-area apex. BLACK now has a chance to hide a disc near the 8/7 line and the vertical 8/8 line. See FIGURE 21.

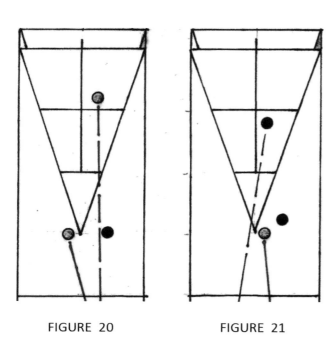

FIGURE 20   FIGURE 21

Hiding Places:

Shuffleboard is a game of "Hide and Seek". Everyone has to be on the lookout for hides. Beginners often fail to recognize a hide because the disc may belong to the opponent.

The advantage of a "discovered/successful" hide: You get 5 discs in lieu of 4. Remember, the hide favors the player that gets there first!

Example of a hide: Middle of the game, YELLOW disc to shoot. BLACK is on the board with a high 8, a deep 10 and a weak St. Pete near the apex of the 10.

A. Try a combination shot: hit the 10 into the 8 and they go off the board, your disc also goes off.

B. Try to put the opponent's high 8 into the kitchen and try to stick. YELLOW, if successful, has two (2) protected discs and a BLACK in the kitchen. Not too bad! See FIGURE 22.

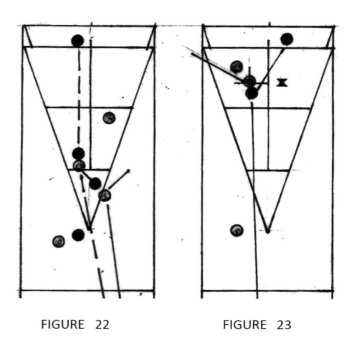

FIGURE 22   FIGURE 23

Keep looking ! A good place to hide is in The corner of the 7-area. Protect the 7 with a St. Pete slightly off, towards the outer edge. Place a disc on the "X" near the 7. See FIGURE 23. The shot is <u>difficult</u>, but with practice it is easy.

BLACK tries a combination shot to clear the board. BLACK's shot hits the disc at "X" and glances off, missing the 7-disc and into the kitchen for a minus 10, or snuggles up to the "X" if the shot is too slow. See FIGURE 23.

BLACK puts up a Tampa which is to the right of its correct position. Try placing a YELLOW disc into the 7-area corner.

BLACK has a direct hit to the YELLOW 7, or BLACK may put a disc in the 8-area to block the YELLOW 7.
BLACK may put a disc in the 8-area to block the YELLOW 7. See FIGURE 24.

HIDING PLACES:

Hiding Places:

One of the best places to hide! BLACK puts a Tampa on the BLACK side of the apex of the 10.

YELLOW puts a disc in the 10-area behind the Tampa for a hide. Very good when the BLACK hammer fails. See FIGURE 25.

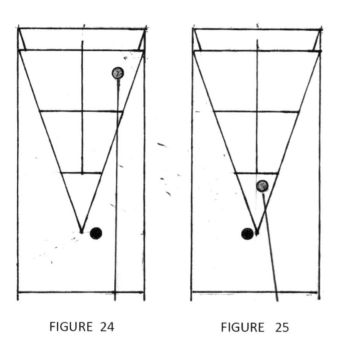

FIGURE 24   FIGURE 25

Hides, End Game:

As in <u>Hide and seek,</u> a hide (sneak) is a shot that is protected in the 7-playing area behind the St. Pete or Tampa by either YELLOW or BLACK.

Hide, is a much used shot in shuffleboard. A hide makes or breaks a game, depending on how well you hide. The strategy for a successful hide:

A. Do not go on the board to hide when you are ahead.
B. Do not play kitchen bait when you are ahead.

Proper kitchen play, does not place bait on the board when it isn't required. When you are ahead, don't <u>risk</u> being put in the kitchen or snuggled.

Beginning players are instructed to hide and get ahead to put pressure on the opponent. If you routinely take unnecessary risk with a hide you will give the game away.

Fake Hide:

The Fake Hide: Place your disc wide and low, near the 8/7 line or as near as possible, but <u>outside</u> of the 7-playing area and partially protected by a St. Pete.

A fake hide is often unrecognized as a hide and is allowed to stay on the playing board without revealing your strategy. See FIGURE 26.

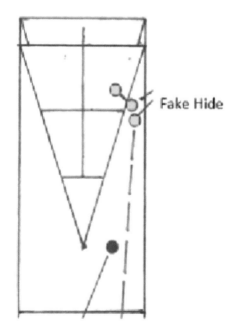

FIGURE 26

Hides, End Game:

When do you need a fake hide?

A. The opponent has the hammer and you need a score from a hide to keep up.

B. When your opponent can go out with either hammer and you need to score a 7 to win.

C. If you have the hammer and need an extra score, try a conventional hide with the third disc. If the hide is good, score with the hammer for a double score.

Every game is a gamble and with many opportunities to take a "Chance". Plan how you want to play, when it doesn't go as planned "CLEAR".

Many players try to "kitchen" and often they are good at it. You will need to govern your play accordingly. A few clues to identify traits of a kitchen player:

A. The player in the practice round, puts all of the 4-practice discs into the 7-area.

B. The player tries to put the opponent's disc into the kitchen regardless of the need.

The End Game: The value of the hide.

A. Your score is 71, a hide score of 7 = (71+7), Your opponent is at 67, they need to kitchen the 7 or clear the 7, or score 2-discs. Even a 10 will not win.

B. Your score is 70, hide score of 7 = 77 (70+7), Your opponent is at 67, they must score a 10 to tie. A 10 is a difficult shot, if they score the game is still on.

C. Your score is 69, you make a 7 = 76 (69+7), The opponent needs a 10 to win. Not an easy shot, but possible.

D. The score is 68, you make a 7 = 75 (68+7),

Your opponent needs an 8 to tie, or a 10 to win, A tough decision.

E. Your score is 67, you make a 7 = 74 (67+7), your opponent needs an 8 to win. Your 7 is no good, you need a high 10 in lieu of a 7 to win.

Decisions, Decisions, Decisions, what a 7 will do for you!!

CLEARING DISCS:

Clearing:

Clearing opponent's discs from the playing area is an important part of the shuffleboard game. To clear: Both the opponent's disc and the cue disc MUST clear the playing area and go off the court, preferably into the gutter. The player that *sticks* the least has the best chance to win. Why a cue disc will stick? See Figure 27.

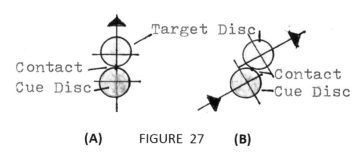

(A)   FIGURE 27   **(B)**

If the cue disc A or B makes a direct hit with the Target disc, regardless of travel speed, or the cue disc is shot too slow it will stick.

If the cue disc strikes the target disc off the centerline the two (2) discs will deflect 90 degrees. For the point of contact see Figure28.

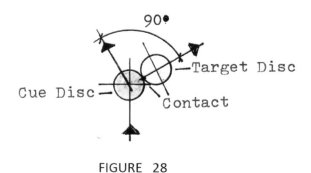

FIGURE 28

To correct unsuccessful clearing of discs you need to aim better and shoot harder.

To shoot harder may cause control problems. Many players fly their arm slightly sideways when shooting hard, trying to miss or stick. If they have the hammer, after shooting too hard, they try to score with the hammer, clear softly and leave discs in the playing area. Practice, practice, is the best cure.

To clear properly, draw an imaginary line from Head to Foot through the center of the playing court, called the Longitudinal Centerline.

YELLOW player: any discs on the **left** side of the Longitudinal Centerline are cleared from spot # 2 (in the starting area). See Figure 29.

YELLOW player: any discs on the *right* side of the Longitudinal Centerline are cleared from spot # 1 (in the starting area). See Figure 30. The opposite is true for the **BLACK** player.

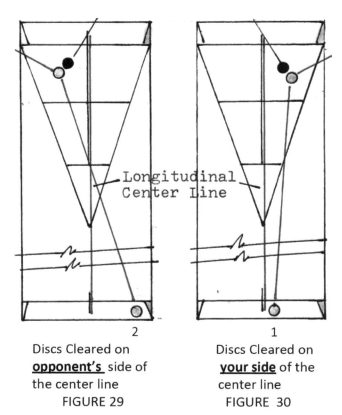

2

Discs Cleared on **opponent's** side of the center line

FIGURE 29

1

Discs Cleared on **your side** of the center line

FIGURE 30

CLEARING DISCS:

Clearing:

What to do about misses? When careful aim does not correct the problem, try reversing the starting spots. The aim is still to the outside of the target disc.

On a drift court, aim slightly away from (instead of into the drift) the center or slightly inside of the Target disc and let the drift provide the deviation.

When you are clearing well, you begin thinking this is easy, fail to concentrate, change your delivery routine, etc. This is a lack of discipline. Success depends upon effective clearing of the playing area to win.

Disc in the Kitchen: What to do??

You are in the kitchen, should you try and CLEAR your disc or wait a turn and see what your opponent does? Options:

A. Try to clear your disc and you do. You are now one (1) less disc to use against your opponent.

B. Try to clear your disc and you Stick. You are now two (2) less discs to use against your opponent.

C. Would it be better to try and hide a disc in the 7 or 8 for a minus 3 or 2 in lieu of a minus 10? You need to look at the score board to determine your next shot before shooting.

Your opponent has the hammer and they are in the kitchen. What should you do?

Strategy: Place a disc in the 7-area, on the opposite side , as far away from the opponent's kitchen disc as possible. This may not be the best play. Why?

Do you need to increase your score or reduce the opponents score and how many discs remain?

If your opponent score is 59 or more, block their kitchen with a high 8 which is in line with the kitchen disc.

Remember the game goes to 75, with 16 more points the game is over. Think, and play to win.

BACKSTOPS:

Backstops:

In shuffleboard, backstops placed by the opponent set up several possibilities. They are as follows:

    1. Discs A, B, C and D used as backstops, stick and score, clear each disc.

    2. Discs A, B, C and D into the kitchen and score.

    3. Disc C is a high 7, the cue disc sticks/scores, whereas the next shot by the opponent, will touch the 8/7 line for no score.

    4. Disc B can be "kissed" for a double.

    5. Disc E if it touches the line it is OK, if it does not touch the line the disc must be removed to prevent it being used as a backstop. See the rules governing shuffleboard play. See FIGURE 31.

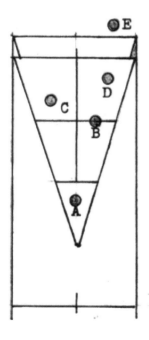

FIGURE 31

Placing High Numbers:

High 10: A difficult shot to make. A low 10 can be used as a backstop to stick/score. If the opponent scores and puts the 10 into the kitchen it's known as an "Up and Down 10."

Use the # 1 shooting position when trying for a 10. Why? Because the hit disc will travel down the middle line for no score. See FIGURE 32.

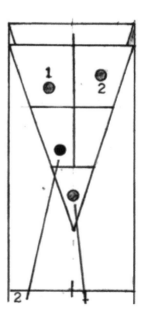

FIGURE 32

High 8: most players prefer the high 8 versus the high 10, because the high 10 is a more difficult shot. To shoot the 8, aim at the mid-point of the 10/8 line. For the shooting position for YELLOW and BLACK, see FIGURE 32.

High 7: Is not used. The 7-area being used for Kitchen-bait prevents the player from using the disc. If there are two (2) 7's in the 7-area, one of the 7's is closer to the 8/7 line than the other, choose the closer 7 and you stick/score. The opponent's next disc will catch a line. See FIGURE 32.

BACKSTOPS:

Snuggles Shot:

YELLOW disc in the 7-area as kitchen bait. BLACK can not afford to fall behind in score. Hence , BLACK snuggles up to the 7 to keep the score even. To snuggle up to the YELLOW disc the player needs a delicate touch.

If BLACK is down in score and YELLOW disc touches the 7/(-10) line. BLACK snuggles up to the 7 for a score. YELLOW can reverse this with the hammer, put BLACK into kitchen to score/win. See FIGURE 33 and 34.

Waste a Shot: Why? To prevent the opponent from using your disc for their advantage.

The best way, shoot the disc so it <u>does not cross the Dead</u> line. Or close to the outer playing edge, it <u>can not</u> be put in the 10-Off.

Never shoot a disc the length of the court with other discs on the board. Play to win.

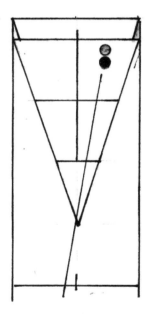

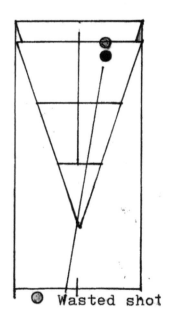

Wasted shot

FIGURE 33   FIGURE 34

COMBINATIONS/CAROMS :

Combinations/Caroms:

The objective of combinations/caroms is to remove a third disc off the board. The difference between these shots are:

1. Combination shot: the cue disc strikes a target disc, <u>the target disc continues on</u> to strike a second target disc.

The Bump shot is an example of a Kitchen shot or a doubles shot. Many chances arise for bunt combinations.

Bump shots generally are low percentage shots because speed and drift of court are hard to control. However ,if you are behind and the opponent has a hide behind your disc, bump in lieu of clearing.

Example of a bump: Three (3) discs close together in a straight line area. This is a kitchen shot with about the same speed required as a single disc kitchen shot. See FIGURE 35.

2. Carom shot: The cue disc strikes the target disc, the <u>cue disc continues on</u> in a different direction to strike a second target disc.

Upon impact, the cue disc hits the target disc at the point of tangency (point of contact) on the circumference of each disc. The discs moves 90 degrees in the opposite direction of each other.

If the direction of the <u>cue disc</u> is changed to the **left**, and the point of contact remains the same, the <u>cue disc</u> will travel further because it has more energy than the target disc.

From physics, a body at rest stays at rest. The target disc is at rest, whereas the cue disc has the speed (energy). If the direction of the <u>cue disc</u> is changed to the **right**, the point of contact remains the same. The <u>target disc</u> will travel further because it has more energy than the cue disc. Why?

From physics, the energy transferred from one body to another is equal and opposite.

To make combinations/caroms shots you need speed and accuracy. See FIGURE 36.

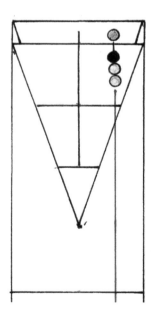

FIGURE 35

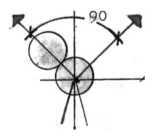

Left   Right

FIGURE 36

Note: See the Enlarged example of the <u>Cue</u> disc striking the <u>Target</u> disc at positions 1,2 and 3.

COMBINATION/CAROMS:

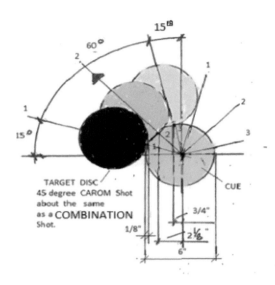

60 Degree RANGE of CUE DISC/TARGET DISC
FIGURE 36 (Enlarged)

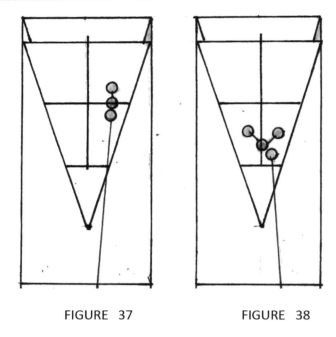

FIGURE 37   FIGURE 38

Doubles: the Horizontal and Vertical double.

A. The **Horizontal double:** About half-way on the 10/8 or 8/7 line with a "<u>kiss</u>" the Cue disc will hit the Target disc and each disc will score. See FIGURE 37.

B. The **Vertical double:** Half-way on the center line, about a foot (1') below the 8/7 line, with a "<u>kiss</u>" from the Cue disc. The Cue disc and the Target disc go 90 degrees to each other, each disc will score.

Doubles leave both discs unprotected which needs to be considered by the player. See FIGURE 38.

With the double, the opponent will try to spoil the scores. This depends upon whether or not the score is important and who has the hammer. Look at the score board first to see the score.

The **Triple:** Scoring three (3) discs, the cue disc plus two (2) others. Difficult shot, seldom a planned shot.

Potential triple shots occur when two (2) of your discs are on the 10/8 and 8/7 line or one disc or two discs are on the centerline and the other disc in the 8-area. See FIGURE 39 and FIGURE 40.

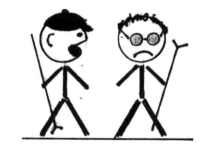

SCORE a TRIPLE ??   Why Not !!

COMBINATION/CAROMS:

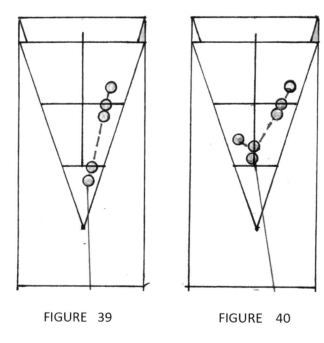

FIGURE 39   FIGURE 40

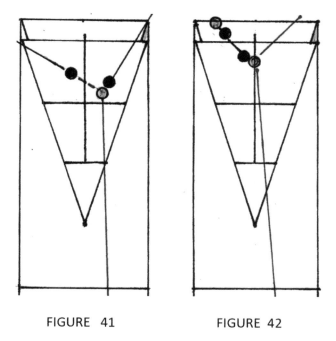

FIGURE 41   FIGURE 42

Caroms:

Caroms: This shot has a greater chance for success when the cue disc glances to one side in lieu of the target disc. Why? Speed (energy) is required to make this shot a success. The cue disc hits the first target disc which absorbs most of the energy and leaves only a small amount of speed (energy) in the cue disc to make the shot good.

Remember, when the cue disc hits the target disc at 45 degrees the success of a combination shot versus a carom shot are nearly equal.

Fundamental Principal: A combination shot leaves the opponent's disc on the board. A carom shot leaves the player's disc on the board. See FIGURE 41 and FIGURE 42.

Glance Shot: an incomplete carom shot is another way to hide a disc.

Example: YELLOW disc on the 8/7 line and BLACK has a disc in the high 7-area. The cue disc hits the BLACK disc and <u>glances</u> off to the left for a hide behind the YELLOW disc on the 8/7 line. The distance between the YELLOW 8/7 and the BLACK 7, 18 inches +/-. This example occurs often. See FIGURE 43.

For another example of a typical glance shot see FIGURE 44.

Practice these shots, they help you to win.

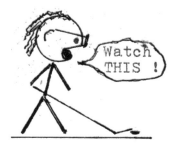

GLANCE SHOT !!

COMBINATION/CAROMS:

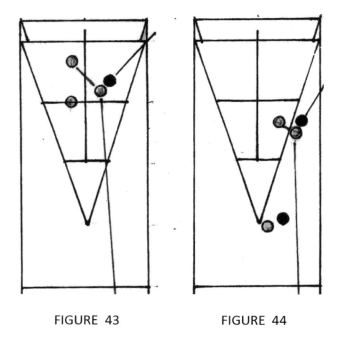

FIGURE 43   FIGURE 44

Combination/Caroms are used as High Speed clearing shots which cause the Target disc to carom into a hidden disc and clear the board.

When to use a Combination/Carom disc to clear?

A. You are ahead and the plan is to clear the board of your opponent's discs.

B. A Combination shot at Kitchen speed when your opponent score is 59 or more , has the hammer and ready to go out.

Combination/Carom shots are LOW percentage shots and only used for specific conditions.

In regular play, when you "see" the opponent's hidden disc and it is **NOT** totally visible, it is very difficult to clear the disc from the board.

The RULE: Use a high speed Combination/Carom take-out shot when the hidden disc is **NOT** visible.

STRATEGY:

Shuffleboard Game:

Shuffleboard game: A series of plays, planned to win the game. To do this: 4-players (doubles) shoot 8-frames from the Head, 8-frames from the Foot in a 16 frame game, or a score of 75, whichever is first. In a point game the score goes to 75.

YELLOW starts first, plays the odd discs, # 1, 3, 5 and 7. BLACK plays the even discs, # 2, 4, 6 and 8.

The Strategy:

(A) Play **Offense**, score points and win the game.

(B) Play **Defense**, keep opponent from scoring points and win the game.

YELLOW starts; Takes the offense, by creating a hide, place a **St. Pete**, otherwise BLACK would clear the board. You want to hide the # 3 disc behind the St. Pete. **BLACK's** # 2 disc clears the board.

Trial and error time! Try the same thing over again. BLACK's # 4 disc clears the board. No Luck! What to do? Place a **Tampa** with disc # 5. BLACK's # 6 disc hits the Tampa and sticks! Lady Luck is Good! Now the YELLOW disc # 7 can hide in the 7-area behind the Tampa. The shoe is on the other foot. The BLACK hammer (disc # 8) can clear the hide and score, or leave the YELLOW 7 and score a 10/8 or 7 on the YELLOW side of the board. Decisions, decisions, what a game!

The first frame is over, now the second frame starts with the YELLOW Foot. The Strategy for YELLOW Foot the same as YELLOW Head. Trial and error, see what happens, and play accordingly. Don't forget your best friend, the Score Board!

In Shuffleboard, defensive strategy does not exist. Why? When a player is behind, they have to become offensive and set up bait to put the opponent into the "kitchen" to reduce the score and keep the game alive. This is an extreme offensive strategy.

Defensive blocks may be used to prevent the other player from scoring, but this is not scoring.

The Game Plan: In 3-parts, the opening, the middle game and the end game.

The play of the game, disc by disc as follows:

Disc # 1: (A) Set up a St. Pete/Tampa or (B) go on the board. If the player is ahead or even with the opponent they should place disc # 1 as a St. Pete or Tampa. The use of disc # 1 does not vary much.

When the player is behind and the opponent needs one score to win, kitchen bait should be set and cleared or clear the next 6 shots, plus a good hammer to score for the win. Hard work and a difficult task.

Disc # 2: When disc # 1 is correctly placed as a St. Pete or Tampa the opponent will clear with disc # 2, or place a block on the board to prevent disc # 3 to be placed for a hide behind disc # 1.

Clearing is always better than blocking, because player of disc # 1, has to set up once more.

Disc # 3, 4 and 5: continue to be used as played in the first 3 shots. The player of these discs needs to be alert to take advantage of any errors the opponent makes to hide without giving up a free score.

Disc # 7: is of no use if the board is clear: used best as a hide. Disc # 4 used to clear off possible doubles, whereas disc # 3 or # 5 used to protect them. If disc # 3 is shot as a hide and stops on a line, disc # 4 used to block disc # 3 to prevent the player from a second chance to hide a score behind the St. Pete or Tampa.

Disc # 6: If the score is even or ahead and the board is clear, disc # 6 can be a plus or a minus. If the board is clear, disc # 6 should not be used as a guard. If the player has an unprotected disc on the board, use disc # 6 as a guard. If the player is behind in score

STRATEGY:

and the board is clear, disc # 6 should be used as kitchen bait.

Disc # 7: Main use is to hide for a score, also to reduce the opponent's chance to score with the hammer. In various places disc # 7 can serve as a block, the positions are: See FIGURE 45.

Position A or B: Not a big distraction to the hammer, always a chance to nip the block and miss the target.

Position C: Good block if the court drifts, do not place as a backstop for a 10 on the 10/8 line.

Position D and E: High numbers, 10 or 8, when the player is behind in score.

Position F: Corner 7 shot, better if a guard is near G.

Do not forget to consider placing # 7 disc into the 10 area behind the Tampa.

Disc #8 Strategy:

1. Clear the board and score the last shot with the hammer. The hammer, very valuable, most players will not take risks, but shoot for a simple shot to score.

2. If the opponent has an unguarded scoring disc on the board, spoil the disc and score.

3. If you are far behind, try a kitchen shot and a score even if the disc is on the line.

4. If there is a **pigeon** (disc on the 10-Off line) use the hammer to kitchen the disc or clear. See FIGURE 45.

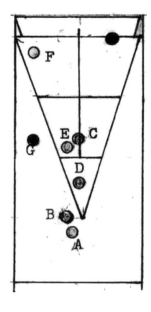

FIGURE 45

The End Game: In shuffleboard it's the most difficult. Why? Now the score board /discipline/ psychology and opportunities enter into the game.

For a point game, the important score to remember is 75 and what score is required to win. In a frame game, which has 16 frames or 75, which-ever is first, keeps the players mentally sharp to the end.

What is the Magic Circle?

In a 75 point game the **Magic Circle** score is as follows:

Score is 57, requires a (10 + 8)=18 + 57 = 75
Score is 59, requires a (8 + 8)=16 + 59 = 75
Score is 60, requires a (8 + 7)=15 + 60 = 75
Score is 65, requires a (10)   =10 + 65 = 75

The importance of these scores in a doubles game, each YELLOW/BLACK have two (2) hammers. Each play two (2) half rounds without a hammer.

The advantage goes to the side which has a score of 60 + in the same round they have the hammer. Hence, it is better for the opponents that are not in the

STRATEGY:

Magic Circle and do not have the hammer, to play carefully, keep the score down and wait for their turn.

In a frame game, the strategy is the same, except the players must keep in mind the exact number of hammers left in the game. In a point game the players must estimate the number of hammers each will need to win.

The game is not over till the last disc is shot. Remember! **Lady Luck** always has a hand in a shuffleboard game, always keep a winning attitude.

The End Game for Fun!!!

The importance of the Score Board, assume the last 2-frames of a 16 frame game. YELLOW Head (doubles) has the hammer, BLACK has a disc in the 7-area and a good deep 10. What is the best shot for YELLOW ?

STRATEGY:

The End Game: (Example)

Assume 3-different games, the score for game (A) 57-59, (B) 59-60 and (C) 60-65.

The score board

	A		B		C	
Beginning of the 15-frame	Y	B	Y	B	Y	B
1. Clear the 10	57	66	57	67	60	72
2. Clear the 7	57	69	57	70	60	75
3. Clear the 7/score 7	64	69	66	70	67	75
4. Clear the 10/score 10	67	66	69	67	70	72
5. Clear the 7/score 7	64	69	66	70	67	75
6. Kitchen the 10	57	66	59	67	60	72
7. Kitchen the 10/score 10	67	66	69	67	70	72

A. Frame 2, 3 and 5 a win for BLACK.
B. Frame 4 or 7 is the best play, because YELLOW foot has the hammer, clear the board for the last shot with an 8 or 7 and win.

Example   # 3

See Figure 46 for a glance shot, (Frame # 4).

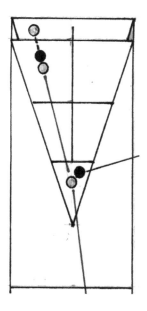

FIGURE 46

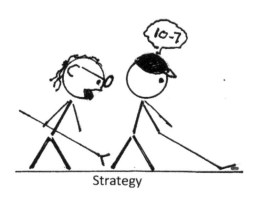

Strategy

STRATEGY:

Playing shuffleboard you often hear, "Don't rush the game," or He/She tried to rush the game.

The score is 71 and what often happens!

1. Playing doubles, the score is 71 and you can try to hide a score when the opponent has the hammer, go out and win. Sometimes Yes, sometimes NO. The opponent puts you in the kitchen, back to 61 and you will need to score 2-discs to go out.

2. If you are the <u>Foot</u> and the score is 71, a hide may give you a win, but a kitchen puts it back to 61. You can still go out with 2-7s when you have the hammer.

3. If you are the <u>Head</u> a hide is not to your advantage, <u>it's rushing the game</u>. Why? If the opponent puts you in the kitchen, you are back to 61, your partner may try to make up the lost 10 and get themselves placed in the kitchen and you are now at 51. You now need 3-discs to win.

4. If your opponent is at 69 and you are at 40 +/- You MUST shoot a 10. The psychology of a 10 may encourage the opponent to make a mistake. It's worth a try.

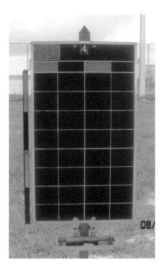

STORY TELLER !!

MODULAR SHUFFLEBOARD:

Modular Shuffleboard: by Wilbur L. Estes, published by Wilbur L. Estes, Copyright 1995 is a complete and definitive treatise to play shuffleboard the Modular way. My thanks, gratitude, to Mr. Estes for his explanation and knowledge of shuffleboard and the way to play the Modular System.

Conventional shuffleboard (doubles) is a point or frame game to 75, a straight line from zero (0) to 75. As the game continues and the score is between 28 to 41, the team with a score of 41 is closest to 75, therefore ahead. However, when the score is 58 to 60 experienced players know who is ahead and what they need to do.

Under t**he Modular System:** when you are in the same or higher bracket and have the **Hammer** at the **Head** of the court, you are ahead. Why? You are at least one scored disc closer to 75 than your opponent.

When you play the Modular System and Game Plan, and execute well, you will have the Hammer when you are 59 or above.

Your team has the hammer, you only need to score two (2) discs to win, [59 +(8+8)=75]. Each partner needs only to clear and score their hammer.

The heart of the Modular System is the Score Bracket. A Module is made up of 16 points which is called a **Bracket**. The brackets are as follows:
- 75 - 16 = 59
- 59 - 16 = 43
- 43 - 16 = 27
- 27 - 16 = 11

You need to remember: **1 1—27—43—59**.

In a 75 point game, you are "Climbing the Stairs" one step at a time. See Figure 47.

Think of the score **Brackets** as stairs to climb. Each bracket is 16 steps to the next bracket. **NOTE:** the first bracket starts with a **minus 5** which is **11 (16-5),** In lieu of zero (0) as in a conventional game. The next bracket is 11+16= 27. Why? Because the

brackets were calculated down from 75, making 11, not 16 the lower limit of the first bracket.

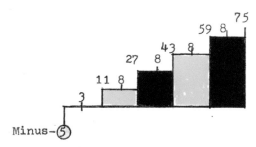

SCORE (Brackets) = 16 Points/Step
FIGURE 47

Many players use "**45, 60 and out**" as a mark to be concerned and play accordingly. If you are at 51, the opponent has the hammer, they may let you score an 8 and get to 59.

At a score of 60, a 7 + 8 will win. However, for those that consider 60 the danger point and allow their opponent to reach 59, making it possible for you to go out with two (2) 8's.

In the first bracket 11, The opponent could go out with a score of 15 + four 7's (28) + four 8's (32)=75, versus 11 + eight 8's (64)=75. The opponent to go out from a 10 requires 9 discs.

Game Plan -- Things to Remember!!

You are ahead -- Have the Hammer
1. Clear the board, keep it clean. Score with your hammer.
2. Hide a score, if you are below 43.
3. Don't try to hide another. Cover your good disc. Score with your hammer.
4. Score with your hammer. Don't chase unless, the opponent's disc is Game Point.
5. Don't block opponent's kitchen. Place a Low 7 on the opposite side, as far away from their kitchen as possible, unless you are 52 or more.
6. Shoot hard, to clear both opponent's 7, and your kitchen, only your hammer is left, try to transfer.

You are ahead – Opponents have the Hammer
MODULAR SHUFFLEBOARD:

MODULAR SHUFFLEBOARD:

1. Set a St. Pete, hope the opponent sticks.
2. If opponent sticks, set another, hope they stick.
3. If opponent sticks, hide, if you are below 43.
4. If opponent goes on the board, clear. Limit them to one score with their hammer.
5. If opponent clears all three of your St. Pete's, block the Point of the 10.

You are Behind – Have the Hammer

1. Clear the first two discs.
2. Bait, Low 7 with your third disc.
3. If the opponent kitchens, try to transfer.
4. If opponent sticks, try to kitchen.
5. If opponent missed, score your hammer.
6. If you miss opponent's St. Pete and they score, try a combination at kitchen speed.
7. Don't block opponent's Kitchen. Score a low 7 on the opposite side-as far away from their kitchen as possible, unless they are at 59 or more.
8. If the opponents are at 68, at the **Foot**, and you can out point them, try a Suicide Alley with your **third** disc.

You are Behind -- Opponents have the Hammer

1. Set a St. Pete (Hope they stick).
2. If opponent clears, set another, hope they stick.
3. If opponent goes on the board-clear it off.
4. Block a Double with your last disc – clear if possible Game Point.
5. **Third Disc**. If you can't hide and opponents are not to 50 or 66, place a **Halfway -8.**
6. Don't block opponent's kitchen. Score a Low 7 as far away as possible _except_ when they have a score of 59, or more. Then score an 8, almost in line with their kitchen.

Halfway – 8:

Place the Halfway – 8 on the opponent's side, a little less than halfway into the 8-area. A difficult shot, but necessary. Why? It's hard for the opponent to clear the disc. If the opponent sticks, they will leave 6 to 9 inches of space for you to hide a high 8. If you kitchen their shot, your high 8 may be a block for their kitchen.

What can the opponent do?

1. They can try to transfer your 8 or kitchen. Opponent may miss the transfer, or the kitchen, or give-up a 7, and still be off minus 10.

2. Your opponent is in the kitchen. They could try to take out their kitchen, miss and your 8 is good, they will be a minus 10. See Figure 48.

The Reinforced Hide:

When your opponent clears the board, sometimes their cue disc will roll for a **partial hide**. You choose to reinforce the opponent's disc by placing your disc next to theirs. Why? The reasons are as follows:

1. Your opponent has the hammer, you are behind, you plan to hide with your third disc. Until then you have to stay off the board.
2. You have the hammer and are behind, you plan to hide on your third disc. Until then you have to stay off the board.
3. Your opponent has the hammer, you are ahead, you want the opponent to clear, keep them from setting up their own play.
4. You are trying to create the illusion of setting up a hide without taking an unnecessary risk. The reinforcement being "obvious," the opponent clears the board. See Figure 49.

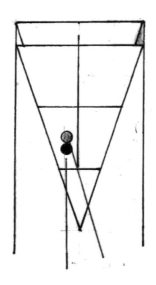
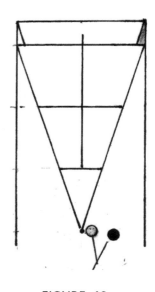

FIGURE 48   FIGURE 49

PRACTICE :

Beginning Practice:

Practice: Repeated performance for the purpose of learning. The beginning player needs to practice two (2) things (A) distance and (B) aim.

A. **Distance:** Practice shooting simple shots to the 7 and 8-area with a delivery that is comfortable for you. Using a <u>Right Hand-Left-Foot</u> or a <u>Right-Hand Right- Foot</u> delivery if right handed.   The opposite if left handed.

B. **Aim:** After the beginner has developed reasonable control of the delivery, they need to practice shots which require more precision. The best shots to practice are those required to start the game. The shots required to start the game are as follows:

1. The <u>YELLOW disc</u>, place a St. Pete on the opponents side of the board.

2. <u>Hide</u> a YELLOW disc behind the St. Pete in the 7-area.

3. <u>Clear</u> off the YELLOW St. Pete with a BLACK disc. <u>Both discs</u> go off the board.

4. <u>Replace the vacant St. Pete</u> position with a BLACK disc.

5. <u>Test</u> the quality of the BLACK St. Pete by trying to spoil the hidden YELLOW disc with a BLACK disc.

6. <u>Repeat steps 1 to 5</u> using the BLACK to start the game.

This drill will help you to open/clear and hide with three (3) discs left to try a Tampa, kitchen, hide, bump or a high 10. Practice this drill as often as you can, once or twice is not enough ! See FIGURE 50.

Practice with another player always better than by yourself. Why? With one player at the Head and the other at the Foot, special shots which require a particular set up, can be easily set up each time by the player who is not in the act of shooting.

To play off a Tie Game: The Florida Shuffleboard Association, Rules and Regulations, October 1, 2010, are as follows:

D–Scoring 4: If a tie game results at game point or over, play is continued in regular rotation of play, until two (2) full rounds in doubles or one (1) full round in singles are completed. At that time the side with the higher score wins, even if it has less than 75 points or the number of points specified as game points. If the score is tied again, play continues as outlined above.

A tie occurs only at game point, or above. The play continues in regular rotation, from when the tie occurred. Therefore, if the game <u>is tied at the Foot</u>, the tie breaker starts at the <u>Head</u>. If the game is tied when played <u>from the Head</u>, the tie breaker starts at the <u>Foot.</u>

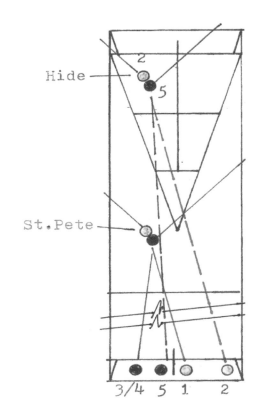

FIGURE 50

PRACTICE:

Practice: Good habits and practice drills make shuffleboard playing enjoyable and fun to do.

Before starting to practice always check to see if the discs are waxed. Nothing is more frustrating than discs that "drag and die".

If you play tournaments you get 2-discs for speed and 4-discs for practice when you shoot YELLOW. When you shoot BLACK you get 2 discs for speed and 4-discs for practice.

If you do not enter tournaments it's still a good habit to practice as outlined above. They say, PRACTICE! PRACTICE! PRACTICE!

Several ways to practice with the 4-discs. They are:

A. With the YELLOW discs in the shooter box. See CHAPTER 1, FIGURE 2 for the shooter box location spots.

From spot # 1, shoot disc to the opposite side of the centerline to the 7-playing area.
From spot # 1, shoot disc to your side of the centerline to the 7-playing area.
From spot # 3, shoot straight down Suicide Alley along the edge to the 7-playing area. This shows you the drift to the deep corner if you plan to hide a disc here.
From spot # 3, shoot across the centerline towards the extreme opposite corner of the 7-playing area. This shot shows you the drift in this area if you want to sneak behind a St. Pete.

B. With the YELLOW disc in the shooter box.

From spot # 3, shoot disc to the 8-playing area and mark your drift chart and not the speed.
From spot # 3, have your partner place a disc in the St. Pete position, shoot a 7 behind it.
From spot # 1, have you partner place a disc in the Tampa position, shoot a 7 behind it.
From spot # 1, have your partner remove the discs and shoot a 10.

Many players practice a 100 point game for fun before they start. See Chapter 14, Games to 100.

Good Luck, Have fun. Remember, **Shuffleboard, WHY NOT??**

TOURNAMENTS:

Shuffleboard Tournaments: Special rules apply to tournaments that are played under the jurisdiction of the Florida National Shuffleboard Association, Inc., Oct. 1, 2008 and the National Shuffleboard Association, Inc.

Florida Sports Foundation is the official sports promotional development organization of the State of Florida. They promote and develop participatory sports for the senior citizens of Florida.

For Information regarding the Florida Senior State Championships, please contact the Florida Sports Foundation at (850)488-8347 or toll free (865)345-2637, e-mail: games@flasports.com.

To compete in the Florida State Senior Games, athletes must compete at their local level and meet the qualifying standards for their sport. The first five (5) finalists in a qualifying game within an age group are eligible to advance to the State Games.

General Rules;

1. Age Division: for singles competition by the athlete's age as of December 31, 2009. Age divisions for doubles/mixed doubles competition will be determined by the younger of the two (2) players as of December 31, 2009.

The following age categories will apply to both men/women in singles/doubles competition.
50-54/55-59/60-64/65-69/70-74/75-79/80-84/ 85-89/90-95 and 100+.

2. Qualification: shuffleboard requires the athlete to qualify at one of the Sanctioned Florida Local Senior Games Qualifiers.

3. Doubles Partners: Doubles partners who qualify together **do not** have to play together at the Florida Senior Games State Championships. Each partner must have qualified at the Florida Local Senior Games Qualifier in order to compete.

4. Residency: Out of state persons may compete at the Florida Senior Games State Championships if they qualify at a Sanctioned Florida Local Senior Games Qualifier. The Florida Sports Foundation's definition of State's Residence: that State in which the person resides for at least six (6) months out of the year.

5. Professional Athlete: Shall not be eligible to compete in the Florida Senior Games State Championships in the sport in which they are or were a professional until 20 years after the date they last competed as a professional.

Ormond Beach Senior Center is a sanctioned Florida Local Senior Games Qualifier. Several other areas in the State are local qualifiers, with different dates and times, contact the Florida Sports Foundation for information.

The Ormond Senior Games

1. Dates and Times: the games are generally in late October and first week in November. Check the Schedule of Events & Venues for date and time information .

2. How to Register: to register you must complete and return the official registration form. All entries must include a signed waiver and entry fees. All payments (checks/money order) made payable to Ormond Senior Games. All entries must be received by a definite date. For information call (386)235-4788 or e-mail: oevermann@msn.com.

3. Number of sports: as many events as you desire without conflicting times. The registration fees are for a single event, plus an extra fee for 2 or more events.

4. Awards: Gold/Silver/Bronze to first, second and third in each event for each age group. First-Fifth place qualifier will advance to the Florida Senior Games State Championships in Lee County, Florida.

5. Games: The shuffleboard games shall be in accordance with the FSA and NSA rules, except as modified. In Ormond Beach they only play doubles.

TOURNAMENTS:

6. <u>Doubles match:</u> consist of 16 frames, with two (2) wins out of three (3) games. The team with the highest point score at the end of 16 frames wins. Teams will change color after 8-frames. In case of a tie, four additional frames will be played.

7. <u>Each player:</u> will have four (4) discs for practice before the start of each match.

8. <u>2010 or even numbered years is a qualifying year</u> for the <u>National Senior Games (NSG).</u> The NSG's are played every two (2) years and are similar in format to the Florida Senior Games State Championships.

9. The Florida State Championships games will be held in Lee County, the City of Cape Coral, Florida, December 6-14, 2008.

10. All 1st, 2nd and 3rd place winners at the Florida Senior Games State Championships will qualify for the 2009 Summer National senior games.

11. The <u>FSGSC and NSG's:</u> play singles one day and doubles the next day for each age group.

12. The courts for the National Senior Games, played at Stanford University, Palo Alto, California Aug 1-15. 2009, were on roll-out vinyl courts with plastic beads, taped onto a concrete surface.

Tournaments , *Playing the Kitchen!*

The Kitchen (-10) Off is only 18 inches deep, therefore, a difficult target. But there are times when it is necessary to put your opponent into the kitchen. One last shot to turn the opponent's 8 into the kitchen and stick for a gain of 18 points.

In one tournament the difficulty of the kitchen shot was figured out. <u>Only 25%</u> of the deliberate kitchen shots were successful. One (1) in every four (4) tries.

If your opponent is 7 or 8 points from game and you are behind 10 or more, go for the kitchen shot.

Remember, your disc is in a straight line with the opponent's minus 10, which makes you an easy shot for your opponent to use the minus 10 for a backstop.

Tournaments are a great experience for tension/discipline/risk taking and the excitement of the challenge to <u>WIN</u> and take a medal back home.

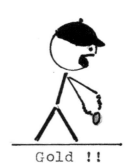

Gold !!

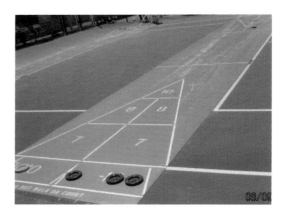

Tournament Courts, Palo Alto, California, 2009

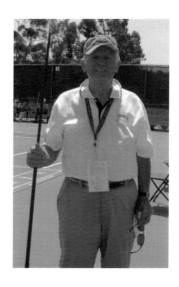

Ready to Play !!
(John Mataya, 2009)

TOURNAMENTS :

How to Play Tournaments:

FORMAT:

1. Athletes shall be divided into pools according to their age division and play a **Round Robin**. If there is only one pool, the first, second and third winners will be determined at the completion of the **Round Robin** (after any ties are broken). If there is more than one pool, the first and second place team/persons in each pool shall advance to a single elimination tournament . A double-elimination tournament shall be played within their age division.

SPORT RULES:

1. All shuffleboard matches shall be conducted in accordance with the FSGSC and NSG rules, except as modified herein.

STRATEGY:

The conventional shuffleboard strategy, the YELLOW player starts the game with a St. Pete for a "Hide and Seek" beginning. The BLACK player would clear the board to make YELLOW set up a St. Pete again, which BLACK would again clear the board. YELLOW would set up a Tampa which BLACK would again clear the board. YELLOW with the 4th disc would try to set a high ten (10) so BLACK would try to kitchen the YELLOW and stick for a good BLACK ten (10) or touch a line for a no-score frame.

Tournament Shuffleboard Strategy: The YELLOW player starts the game with a disc in the high eight (8) or high seven (7) position. BLACK player has the Hammer, may try to clear the YELLOW disc and stick. The game is now "Run and Catch me." Why?

A. The majority of the tournament courts are very fast and sprinkled with silicon beads which makes it difficult to place a disc into the kitchen.

B. Now you are playing a game to 6 frames YELLOW, switch and play 6 frames BLACK. You no longer have the luxury to set up a Hide and Seek. You are into a Run and Catch me game. The player with the Hammer has the best opportunity to score.

C. The player that STARTS the game with BLACK has the advantage because BLACK has the Hammer. When the players switch after 6 frames, BLACK plays the YELLOW discs and has the Hammer in the 12th frame. See Example # 4.

BLACK Player: Starts and Ends with the HAMMER.

EXAMPLE # 4

D. Fast Courts with beads take less effort to propel a disc to the intended target. This type of court favors the player who is patient, observant and accurate in their delivery.

A fast court with beads Is best for a player who "Charts" shots.

Why? As you play on various courts you record the Drift of the court. On fast courts, as the shot disc loses its momentum and comes to a rest it will curl to the low side of the court surface and can easily be observed and recorded. Charting courts takes time, but they pay huge dividends when playing Round Robin Tournaments against a large number of players.

Local players on fast courts have a decided advantage against new players because each player gets only 4 practice shots with each color which makes it difficult to judge speed and drift.

E. Many players use "Speed" to clear the board. They run the risk of making contact with the intended target and sticking or missing the target in lieu of clearing the board. When using speed the body effort and grip tighten which cause the cue disc to miss. The player needs to keep the stroke and delivery the same for every shot. It takes practice and discipline to keep the stroke simple and true.

INTRAMURAL TOURNAMENT:

Intramural Tournament Schedule:

INTRAMURAL Tournament: A very good way for players to get to know everyone that plays shuffleboard on different days and time of the week. Why? Generally, in league play a person signs up for a specific day and time that they want to play. They may play a whole season in their time slot and not meet other players. Only at a general meeting, to vote and select new officers for the next season do they see and meet other players.

Intramural Play gives all the players a chance to meet and play each other and to determine which day and time slot has the best group of players. "Bragging Rights," does a lot of good to promote and encourage others to play and enjoy the game of shuffleboard.

Intramural Tournament Schedule for example is a follows:

1. The League has 6-courts to play on, 7-days per week.
2. The number of players eligible; 4 persons x 6 courts = 24 players per time slot.
3. Time slots: Mon/Tue/Wed/Thur/Fri=5 times.
4. Times to play: (EXAMPLE) Mon @9 A.M./Tue @1 P.M./Wed @1 P.M./Thur @9 A.M./Fri @ 9 A.M.
5. Each time slot has a Captain and a Co-Captain
6. Number of Eligible players in league: 24 players /court x 5 time slots = 100 people.
7. Minimum 2, maximum of 4 players travel from each time slot to another time slot, see the schedule.
8. Play 3-games, 16 frames, 1st game YELLOW, switch and play 2nd game BLACK. Players at the Head, for the 3rd game color decided by coin toss or by lagging for color, one (1) lag for practice, 2nd lag for real.
9. Play Doubles with 2 at Head and 2 at Foot. The Home time slot to start and play Yellow.
10. Before play, each player shall have 4-practice shots per color. The 3rd game no practice shots.
11. If one team has one (1) player, He/She may walk back and forth.

12. The captains of each time slot keep the record of win/loss for each game played and submit results to the official in charge of the Intramural Tournament.

13. At the end of the 4-week tournament the winning team shall be given a certificate and photograph.

The SCHEDULE: Example #5

Week					
Monday @9 A.M.	Fri	Thu	Wed	Tue
Tuesday @1 P.M.	Mon	Fri	Thur	Wed
Wednesday @1 P.M.	Tue	Mon	Fri	Thur
Thursday @9 A.M.	Wed	Tue	Mon	Fri
Friday @9 A.M.	Thur	Wed	Tue	Mon

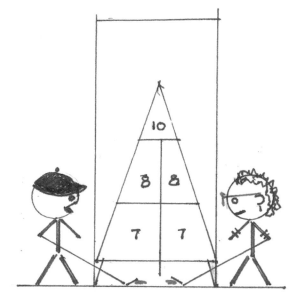

COMMON GROUND !!

GAMES to PLAY:

Ten Pin Game:

Shuffleboard game played with two (2) wooden bowling pins placed at the intersection of the 10/8 line and the vertical 8/8 line. See Figure 51 for the **exact** location.

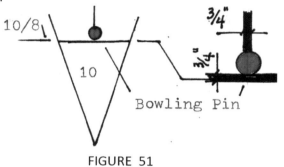

FIGURE 51

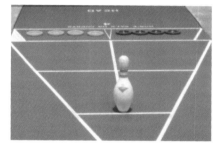

Location of the Bowling Pin

The purpose of the bowling pin is to make the game more interesting by deducting a minus ten (10 Off) the score each time the bowling pin is knocked over by a shot disc. Also the shot disc is removed from the playing field. The game is in two (2) parts as follows:

A.   A score of 65 is required before a player, YELLOW or BLACK, **can start play for part B.**
B.   To end the game, the color with 65 points must go out on a perfect 10.

When the bowling pin is knocked over, it shall be reset, close to its original position. Also, the disc which is shot, shall be removed from the playing area. The person playing YELLOW, keeping score, shall place a small "x" in the frame of the player who shot the disc. The frame continues until all the discs of that frame are shot and scored. It is possible for a player to have a minus 10 from being in the kitchen, plus knocking over

the bowling pin for a minus 10, for total of minus 20 for that frame.

When the side which has 65 points, knocks over the bowling pin, their score goes back to 55 and they have to remake up the required 10 points to be eligible to play again and end the game on a perfect 10.

The Game Plan and Strategy which is the **start, middle** game and the **end game;**

A.   The *opening start:* is similar to a typical start by YELLOW, either a St. Pete or a Tampa to create a hide. Or use the bowling pin for a hide, place the disc in the 7-area on the YELLOW side near the vertical 7/7 line and the 7/(-10) line.

B.   The **middle** game: is conventional shuffleboard, except once a player, YELLOW or BLACK, reaches a score of 65, their score stops and is listed as 65 by the score keeper, but the opponent's score is continued to be counted until they reach a score of 65.

The player without the hammer can often bait by placing a disc in the 10-playing area, hoping the opponent will try to get the 10 out, shoot too hard and knock the bowling pin over for a minus 10. The hammer for score and the kitchen shot to delay the game are used to get to 65 first.

C. The **end game:** starts when a player has a score of 65. They need a perfect 10 to win.

The **game** is now "**ON.**" Your opponent has 65 and the hammer. Typical play, place a disc at the apex of the ten (10) to prevent the 65 player to score and win the game. Instead, place a score in the 8 or 7 area for a score. Why? Because all of your next efforts will be to keep the 65 player from going out. The 7 or 8 will help build up your score in an effort to get to 65.

You have the hammer and 65. Place the first disc at the apex of the (10). The opponent knocks your disc out. Place a second disc on the apex of the (10), your opponent knocks your disc out. Place your third disc as near the slant line of the 10-playing area as near as possible. Your opponent sets a disc near the apex of the (10). With a carom shot try to put your third disc

GAMES to PLAY:

Into the 10 area to win.

The Ten Pin game does not end after 75 or 16-frames, it continues until a player goes out on a perfect 10. Some games may take an hour or more to play.

This game is excellent practice for making carom shots to clear discs for the 10-area, setting up blocks, scoring 10's so your opponent can knock the disc out and the bowling pin down for a minus 10. A large number of shots used in this game will be a big asset in playing conventional shuffleboard.

Rotation Game:

The Rotation game is played with three (3) players and is played as follows:

Each player enters their name on the score board directly above each column as follows:

A's name above the **First** column ; **B**'s name above the **Second** column: **C**'s name above the **Third** column.

A, YELLOW Head: B, BLACK Head and C goes to the YELLOW Foot. The game starts, with YELLOW as the score keeper. YELLOW/BLACK each shoot, the score for example ends YELLOW 8, BLACK 7.

The YELLOW player "A" goes to the YELLOW Foot and the third person "C" on YELLOW Foot moves over to BLACK Foot, they each shoot back towards the Head. The score for example ends YELLOW 15, BLACK 14. The score on the score board is: A -(8+15)=23, B- blank: C -14.

"C," the BLACK Foot goes to the BLACK Head and the "B" BLACK Head moves over to the YELLOW Head. "B," now the YELLOW Head; C the BLACK Head play and the score for example at the end is B, YELLOW 14 and C, BLACK a minus 10. The score on the score board is: B -(7+14)=21: C-(-10+14)=4.

Example of an 8-frame rotation game.

Score Board

Frame	A	B	C		
1	8	7	-	A/B h = 8	7
2	23	-	14	A/C f = 15 -	14
3	-	21	4	B/C h = 14-(-10)	
4	38	28	-	B/A f = 7 -	15
5	45	-	11	A/C h = 7 -	7
6	-	35	21	C/B f = 10 -	7
7	35	43	-	A/B h=(-10) -	8
8	42	-	29	A/C f = 7 -	8

Example # 6

Each player will have the opportunity to practice the **_low_** drift at the Head and the **_high_** drift at the Foot, as each player rotates.

Court drift favors one player over the other. For example, the court drifts towards the YELLOW side, the BLACK player has the advantage in every game on that court. This is called a "BLACK Court." The opposite is true, if the drift is on the BLACK side it's called a "YELLOW Court."

When a court drifts the player has to compensate for the amount of the drift. The drill is as follows:

A. Determine the aiming-point as if on a "level" court for the target.

B. Choose a new aiming-point for the high side of the target, based on your determination of the amount of drift. Next, shoot the disc.

Also, the player knows that a slow shot drifts further off course than a fast shot. This makes long kitchen shots for discs in the 7-playing area difficult.

All shuffleboard players interested in improving their game should include this game for practice on high drift courts.

GAMES to PLAY:

Game to 100:

Game to 100: played by two persons, one player at the Head and the other player at the Foot. Also, this game can be played by yourself, if you want additional practice for score and kitchen shots.

The game is played using the 10, 8, 7 and the minus 10 playing areas. The game goes 4-frames and the player with the largest score wins.

Example: YELLOW starts the game and keeps the score.

YELLOW Head looks at the board and says, two (2)- 7's plus two (2)- 8's = 30 (14+16). Not bad, go for it! YELLOW scores 30, great start!

BLACK Foot looks at the board and goes for a 10,8, and a 7 which goes into the kitchen (-10), puts another disc for a good 7, for a score of 15.

Frame # 2:
YELLOW Head: 2-7's, 2-8's = 30 (14+16).
BLACK Foot: 10, 7 and 2-8's = 33 (10+7+16).
Frame # 3:
YELLOW Head: 7, 8, and a 7 into kitchen (-10), and another 10 which touches a line, = 5 (7+8-10).
BLACK Foot: 2-7's, 8 and a 10 = 32 (14+8+10).
Frame # 4:
YELLOW Head: 2-7's, 8 and a 10 on a line = 22 (14+8).
BLACK Foot: 7, 7 which touches a line, 8, and another 8 which touches a line, = 15 (7+8).

The results of the game are

Frame	Y	B
1.	3 0	15
2.	30	33
3.	5	32
4.	22	15
	87	95

EXAMPLE # 7

If the game ends in a tie the players continue to play until one side wins.

The game can be expanded for the game of kitchen, as follows:

EXAMPLE: BLACK Head shooting area and the BLACK discs, place the discs as follows;

Frame # 1: Place 2- discs in the 7 area and 2-8's in the 8 area.
BLACK Head: 1-7 into (-10)= 10. 3 shots missed.

BLACK Foot: 1-7 into (-10), 1-8 into (-10)= 20, 2-shots missed.
Frame # 2: Place 2-discs in the 10-area and 2-discs into the mid 7-area.
BLACK Head: YELLOW missed all 4-shots = 0.
BLACK Foot: 1-7 into the (1-10)= 10, 3- shots missed.
Frame # 3: Place 2-discs on the vertical line between the 8/8 and 7/7 line, and 2-discs in the 7-area as far apart as possible.
BLACK Head: 1-8 vertical into (-10) =10, 3-shots missed.
BLACK Foot: BLACK missed all 4-shots = 0.
Frame # 4: Place 2-discs on the 8/7 line and 2-discs in the 7-area towards the corner and deep.
BLACK Head: 1-8 into (-10) = 10, 3-shots missed.
BLACK Foot: 1-7 into (-10) = 10, 3-shots missed

The results of the <u>Kitchen</u> game are:

Frame	Y	B
1.	10	20
2.	0	10
3.	10	0
4.	10	10
	30	40

EXAMPLE # 8

This game is excellent practice for each player to work on scoring and trying Kitchen shots on a lot of discs in different locations. It takes patience, discipline and risk to become a better player and win often.

GAMES to PLAY:

Game: *40/out in 10 Frames*

Game 40/out in 10 frames: is the **Perfect** game to play. This game is similar to bowling a score of 300/ grand slam in baseball/pitch a perfect baseball game or a hole-in-one in golf.

The game is played by two (2) players one at the Head and the other at the Foot. The object of the game, make a score of four (4) in each of the ten (10) frames, for a total of 40 points. Similar to shooting "free-throws," in basketball.

The frames are as follows:

1. 7-playing area   4 points
2. 8-playing area   "
3. 10-playing area   "
4. 7-into kitchen   "
5. 8-into kitchen   "
6. 10-into kitchen   "
7. Horizontal-Double   "
8. Vertical-Double   "
9. Bump disc for score/block   "
10. Clear disc from minus 10   "
              Total   40 points

This is the ultimate practice game. A score of 30 to 35 is considered "**excellent,**" **good** from 20 to 25 and less than 20 the player needs more practice.

Each time a disc is shot, the disc is removed from the playing area so the shooter has a clear playing field.

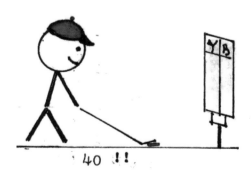

Example: how to score.

Score	Y	Board B
7	3	3
8	3	4
10	2	3
K - 7	2	3
K - 8	1	2
K -10	0	2
Horiz Dbl	2	4
Vert Dbl	1	3
Bump/Block	0	2
Clear (-10)	2	4
	16	30

EXAMPLE # 9

The vertical double range starts at the 10/8 line and goes down to below the 8/7 line about 12 inches. Why? To keep either disc from going into the kitchen. See Figure 52.

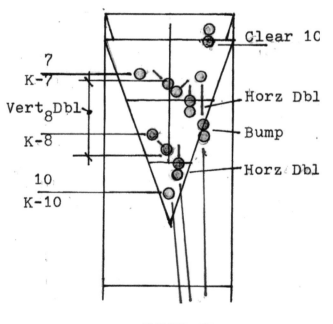

FIGURE 52

44

GAMES to PLAY:

Game: 10-Off before Score Counts

Game: 10-Off before score starts, is a simple game for two (2) players. Both players start at the Head and walk back and forth. Each player YELLOW/BLACK plays one game YELLOW one (1) game BLACK. The third game for color is a toss of a coin.

The object of the game: Each player has to place their disc into the 10-Off area **before** they can begin to count score to win the game.

Once the player, YELLOW/BLACK has a good minus 10, they can start to play a <u>conventional game</u> of shuffleboard for score. The game goes to 75 or number of points at the end of 16 frames, whichever comes first.

The strategy, keep your opponent from placing a disc into the 10-Off area by either blocking or knocking their disc out. Also, try to place your other discs for a good score.

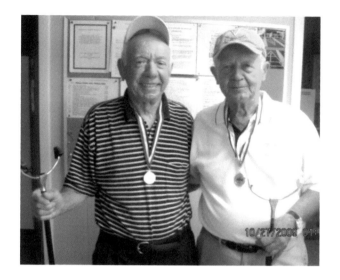

Tony Manzo / John Mataya
Ormond Beach, Fl 2008 (Doubles 80-84) Silver

Tip: place a good disc into the 10-area. Your opponent will have to clear your good 10 to prevent you from getting too far ahead, until they can score a minus 10 and start scoring.

Often you can be 30 to 40 points ahead before your opponent can begin to score. With this advantage your opponent has to use all of the defensive strategies they have to keep the game alive.

This is an excellent game for practicing blocks, knocking discs out of the 10-Off area, shooting 10's and trying to keep the game alive when 50- 40 +/- points behind.

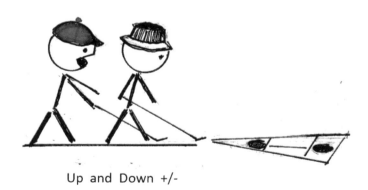

Up and Down +/-

Games are fun and one of the best ways to improve your game. Play often.

GAMES to PLAY:

Game: Turkey Shoot

Shuffleboard Club annual Holiday TURKEY SHOOT . Each Club member has a chance to win a Turkey or other prizes. No fee just play and win.

The date: _M_D_Y,
The Time: _____, A.M.
The Place: _____Shuffleboard Court.
The Event Director_____
Phone #:_____
E-mail: _____

Rules: Each club member that registers will be given a Number on a card which will be returned to the the assistant director upon the completion of their try at winning the First, Second or Third Prize.

The GAME: Each player at the Head of the shuffleboard Court will shoot six (6) discs from the shooter box (ignore the shooter triangle between the YELLOW/BLACK side) at any position they chose.

The color of the disc does not matter.

The discs are shot one at a time, similar to shooting free-throws in basketball. The maximum score possible is 60 (10 x 6=60) for the ½ round from the Head.

The player upon completion of the 6-discs at the Head shall go to the Foot and shoot six (6) discs again.

The maximum score possible is 60 (10 x 6=60) for the ½ round from the Foot. For a grand total of 120 points.

The game continues till there is a First, Second and Third winner.

.

To add a "Joker " to the score: If the player shoots a disc into the minus 10 area, in lieu of a DEDUCT this becomes a PLUS 10 which is added to their score.

Have fun, ENJOY THE FREE HOLIDAY TURKEY!!

SELECTED SHOTS:

Selected Shots:

Beginners frequently ask, what shots should I practice to improve my game?

My selection of shots for beginners or advanced shuffleboard players is as follows:

Using the golf analogy: Play 18 holes of golf, a score of 72. The rules allow 14 golf clubs, from driver to putter. The putter is used for 32 strokes, 40 strokes (72-32) to be used between 13 clubs, one ball and 4-hours +/- to play.

Shuffleboard is a similar game: one (1) cue stick, 8-discs, 4-YELLOW/4-BLACK for a game of 75 or 16 frames, player with the best score wins.

In doubles/singles each side has 8-hammers, 16 frames x 4-discs = 64 shots/ game. 56 shots (64-8) for the other discs used to score/extend the game, which takes 1 to 1½ hours to play 3-games.

In order of preference the shot vocabulary as follows:

1. *Hammer*, for the last shot and score.
2. *Kitchen*, reduce the opponent's score and extend the game.
3. *High 10*, score/bait.
4. *St. Pete*, begin the game.
5. *Tampa*, begin the game/set blocks.
6. *Horizontal Double*, for 2-scores.
7. *Vertical Double*, for 2-scores.
8. *Sucker's Hide*, behind and need a score.
9. *Suicide Alley*, behind and need a score.
10. *Variety of Shots/Scoreboard*, and frame determine choice and type of shot.

The opening game/middle game/ and the end game, require using the above shots to win consistently.

In a 16 frame game, the opening (first 4-frames) require a St. Pete or Tampa. The middle game (next 8-frames), require the use of the Hammer / Kitchen and a variety of shots for score/extend game, etc.

The end game (last 4-frames) depends upon the scoreboard and strategy the player needs to win!

To play shuffleboard it is good to have a strategy, to know whether you are ahead or behind. The Modular System of play, using the brackets (stair steps) at each round of play (Head/Foot) lets you determine your position. Remember the numbers 11, 27, 43, and 59 after each bracket. The end game, with a score of 59 plus two 8's =75, with 2- hammers you win.

Also, you need a variety of shots in the middle game to get ahead or extend the game using hides, blocks, combinations, caroms, bumps and keeping the board clear. The scoreboard sets the stage and the shot that is required for success. Play smart, be smart, good **LUCK !** Keep a positive attitude and yes, Lady Luck does Help. See FIGURE 53.

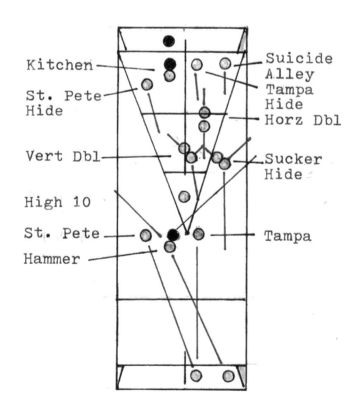

FIGURE 53

SELECTED SHOTS:

Selected Shots:

All shuffleboard instructors rate the Hammer to be the most valuable disc of the four discs required to set-up your play.

The hammer is a positive tool to advance your score towards 75 and win.

Often, the use of the hammer will not produce the desired goal. Your shot will go short or long and more often catch a line for no score.

The hammer is not an automatic shot. You need to treat the hammer as a pressure shot. Establish a "**shot routine**" and practice it like a "**religion**". Take a little extra time, check your delivery stance, check your aim and take the drift into account before you impulsively shoot in the direction of the target.

Game Point Rule:

RULE # 1: Head position, you can see the opponent's disc. **Do NOT** leave the game on the board to go for a win. If the opponent's disc is open**, clear it off**. If you **cannot** see the opponent's disc , go for the win.

RULE # 2: Foot position, If you **cannot** score on your opponent's disc, **leave their disc**. Go for the winning score.

RULE # 3: Do Not chase with the hammer. If your opponent's disc is game, you chase with the hammer. The rule is a reminder to think, do not automatically chase the opponent's hidden disc.

Often the opponent will cover their good disc slightly wide with a slightly deep Tampa halfway down on the outside of the 10. The opponent's good disc is now open for a shot outside of their block. The opponent hopes you will "nick" the Tampa and glance off.

Strategy: The opponent has a hidden disc and only needs to score their hammer.

Often psychology may help. Before you shoot your last shot, examine your hopeless situation in detail. Move your disc around in the shooting box, take several looks at possible shots, look at the score board, take a "second look". You have little chance to rescue the game, the opponent has the hammer. Why this delay?

The longer the delay the more time the opponent may lose their "feel" of the court and miss their hammer.

Shuffleboard, WHY NOT? More head less physical.

Shuffleboard Rules & Regulations
FLORIDA SHUFFLEBOARD ASSOCIATION, INC.
Changes Effective OCTOBER 1, 2008

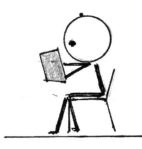

A – Game

1.   The game of shuffleboard is played by either two (2) persons (called singles), or by four (4) persons (called doubles).

2.   The object of the game is to propel discs by means of a cue onto scoring diagram at opposite end of court to score, to prevent opponent from scoring, or both.

B - Equipment

1.   Discs shall be made of composition not less than 9/16" and not more than 1" in thickness, 6" diameter, and not less than 11-1/2 ounces in weight. New discs shall weigh 15 ounces.

Four (4) discs shall be colored YELLOW, four (4) colored BLACK. These eight (8) discs comprise a set. (Other colored combinations may be used, as white, red, blue, etc., as long as there are two contrasting colors). Care should be taken that all discs in a set shall be uniform in weight and thickness.

2.   The cue shall not have an overall length of more than six feet, three inches (6'-3"). No metal part on cue shall touch playing surface of court.

3.   Players shall not be required to play with discs, new or old, that are not in satisfactory condition. Defective discs will be replaced by good discs, if available. Any change of discs must be made before the first (1st) game begins. New discs are not to be used in tournament play, unless thoroughly broken in.

C - Playing Rules
Color Rotation for Main Event and Consolation Final Matches

1.   Player, or team, with lowest line number will play the first game with YELLOW discs, change color and play the second game with BLACK discs. If a third game is necessary, players will shoot for color choices as described in 2c, below, immediately and decide which color they have selected before leaving the court. This decision will be final and may not be changed. Failure to make the decision of color choice before leaving the court, and indicate such choice on the Scoreboard, forfeits this right and gives the color choice to the opponents. [Approved by FSA Board 10/14/2006 and 03/10/2007 and 03-04-2009].

1a.   When beginning a match, before the practice round begins for the first game; each player may shoot two(2) discs only to check the speed of the court. These two (2) speed shots must be taken before any court may be swept and/or beaded. After the first game of a match, if all competitors on a court agree, the court may be swept and/or beaded before the optional speed shots are taken for the second game. There shall be no setups of any kind when taking speed shots.

1b.   Two full rounds of practice on your assigned color are allowed before the first and second games, and no practice is allowed before the third game.

1c.   In doubles, partners shall play on the same color at both ends of the court.

1d.   In doubles, players may change ends once immediately at the conclusion of the practice rounds before the first game begins. Team assigned to the YELLOW discs must decide first whether to change ends or not, and the decision stands for the match, after which the team assigned to the BLACK discs must decide whether to change ends or not, and the decision stands for the match.

2.   Consolation matches will be best two-out-of-three 75-Point games in centerfold tournaments. In District sponsored tournaments, consolation games may be played to 100 points.

2a.   Before practice rounds begin, each player may shoot two (2) discs only to check the speed of the court. There shall be no setups of any kind.

2b.   In 100 Point games, two full rounds of practice with each color are allowed for each player or team before shooting for color choice.

2c.   In shooting for color choice, players must shoot from the Head of the court. In Non-Walking singles, the match at the Foot of the court will shoot for color choice from the Foot of the court. To determine the color choice, any two opposing players (one from each side) each shoot four (4) discs to the far deadline. The players shoot alternately: first YELLOW (or alternate color), then BLACK, then YELLOW, etc. The first three discs of each player are for practice and are removed progressively; the last disc of each player is left on the court. As between these last two discs, the disc nearest the line determines who shall have color choice. The measurement is from center of disc to center of line, EXCEPT if the disc is not touching the line, it shall be measured from the edge of the disc closest to the line to the edge of the line closest to the disc. If the last BLACK disc shot touches or moves the last YELLOW disc, the color choice goes to the player of YELLOW. The last disc of each color shot shall be left in place until inspected by at least one member of each team and the winner agreed upon. If moved, whichever team moved the disc concedes the lag.

3.   To start a game, the YELLOW disc is shot first. Play alternates – YELLOW then BLACK – until all discs are shot. YELLOW shall always be played from the right side of the Head of the court, and left side of Foot of the court.

3a.   ERROR IN COLOR LEAD OR WRONG COLOR PLAYED: Error in color lead or wrong color played shall be corrected if discovered before the half-round is completed; and the half-round shall be played over. If the half-round is completed, the scoring shall be credited to the players making the score, regardless of the color shot, and play continues in the correct order. (The HALF-ROUND is completed when the eighth disc is shot and all discs come to a stop).

3b.   SHOOTING OPPONENT'S DISC: Player shooting opponent's disc; if LIVE disc is not touched, PENALTY – 10-Off, and opponent's disc shall be returned to the starting position and play continued as before the infraction. If a LIVE disc is touched, PENALTY – 10-Off; plus any 10-Offs offender had on the court; good disc of the offender does not count. Opponent's good disc shall be credited to opponent's score (excepting any 10-Offs) and the Half-round shall be played over. The penalties will be annotated on the scoreboard; however, the Half-Round is not complete until the 8th disc has been shot by the correct player.

      If player shoots his or her disc from opponent's respective half, and live disc is not touched: PENALTY -10 Off, that disc is removed from court and play continues. If a live disc is touched, penalty 10-Off, plus any 10-Offs the offender had on the court, other good disc of offender shall not count. Opponent's good disc on court shall be credited to opponent's score EXCEPT any 10-Offs and the frame shall be played over unless game point has been reached by offender's opponent.

3c. In WALKING SINGLES, after all discs are played, completing a HALF-ROUND, the players walk to the other end of court, or Foot of court, and start play with color lead changed to BLACK. The players are to use their own alley to proceed to the other end of the court.

3d. In DOUBLES, after all discs are played at head of court, play starts at Foot or opposite end –YELLOW leading, BLACK following. Color lead does not change until both ends have been played (a ROUND).

3e. All State-sponsored or Statewide Doubles and Walking Singles tournaments shall be 75 Points, best two-out-of-three games, MAIN and CONSOLATION event divisions. All State-sponsored or Statewide Non-Walking Singles shall be best two-out-of-three-games of 16 frames or 75 points, whichever comes first, MAIN and CONSOLATION Event divisions. In tournaments other than the State- sponsored or Statewide events, play may be limited to a specific number of frames, such as 8-12-16 or 20. A FRAME shall be defined to be equal to a Half-Round; every time a score is posted to the scoreboard it constitutes a frame.

In tournaments other than State-sponsored or State-wide events, the third game, if needed, may be 8 (or some other even number) of frames on each color, regardless of score.

In tournaments other than State-sponsored or State-wide, the format of limited frames, such as 16 frames or 75 points, whichever occurs first, is not a violation of the frame limits above and is permitted in Districts which may wish to try the format.

4. Players shall place their four (4) discs within and not touching lines of their respective half of 10-Off area. PENALTY: 5-Off. Penalty not applied to a player until he/she has played a shot.

4a. Discs must be played from the clear from within the respective half of 10-Off area. If disc played touches front or back lines, PENALTY: 5-OFF.

4b. If disc played touches side line, or triangle, PENALTY: 10-Off; offender's disc removed, and opponent credited with any of his/her discs displaced. All displaced discs shall be removed from the court immediately after scoring opponent's displaced discs. Any 10-Offs the offender had on the court that were displaced will be removed before further play and also be deducted from offender's score.

DISC TOUCHING LINES: It is common practice with players to jockey or slide the playing disc backward and forward to see if there is sand which might interfere with disc sliding evenly. No PENALTY is to be called on this practice if lines are touched or crossed while jockeying Disc in motion may cross outside diagonal line.

A disc is played (in the act of shooting) when it is completely in the 7-area. If a disc is touching the farthest dead line, it is in play.

If disc does not reach lag line and is not called dead and is not removed, play should continue and the disc shall be treated as a live disc for that half-round.

5. Players must not touch a foot, hand, knee, or any other part of their body to the court on or over the baseline or extension of the baseline at any time while executing a shot. PENALTY: 10-Off.

6. Players may stand behind baseline extension in the alley between the courts before or while shooting,

but not on adjoining court. PENALTY: 5-Off.

6a. The area between the baseline of the court and on imaginary line, even with the back of the bench, and bounded on the sides by the farthest line of each adjoining alley, should be considered part of the court.

7. In Doubles and non-walking singles, players must remain seated when play is to their end of the court until the last disc has been shot and comes to rest. PENALTY: 5-Off except players can remove dead discs within 8" of baseline, judge discs and retrieve dead discs that have gone onto other courts. In Walking Singles, a player must not cross the baseline to proceed to the other end of the court until all discs are shot and stopped. PENALTY: 5-Off.

8. Players must not leave the court during a game without permission, EXCEPT to gather discs at end of half-round. PENALTY: 10-Off.

8a. No penalty if player leaves court between games. Player may not be gone more than ten (10) minutes. PENALTY: 10-Off. A game is concluded when the referee announces the score, the score is recorded on the scoreboard, and the scores are recorded on the player's card. The referee on the court shall state the time when the game is concluded. Additional penalties may be awarded for further infractions. See Rule C19.

9. Players shall not stand in the way of, or have a cue in the way of, or interfere with, any other players at any time. PENALTY: 5-Off.

9a. Player, after shooting a disc, shall step to the rear of his/her portion of the shooting area with his/her cue in a vertical position in order not to disturb his/her opponent's play. PENALTY: 5-Off.

10. Players shall not touch live discs at any time. PENALTY: 10-Off, plus any 10-Offs the offender has on the board. Other good discs of offender shall not count. Opponent's good discs on the court shall be credited to opponent's score, EXCEPT any 10-Offs, and the half-round shall be played over, UNLESS game point has been reached by offender's opponent. Except, in non-walking singles if a live disc is touched the end shall be played over with no penalty assessed and no score allowed.

11. Players must not talk or make remarks to disconcert opponent's play. PENALTY: 10-Off.

12. Any remark or motion to partner which indicates coaching his/her play is prohibited. PENALTY: 10-Off.

13. Player shooting before opponent's disc comes to rest, PENALTY: 10-Off plus any 10-Offs the offender has on the board. Other good discs of the offender shall not count. Opponent's good discs on the court, prior to the offense, shall be credited to opponent's score, except any 10-Off and the half-round shall be played over, unless game point has been reached by opponent.

14. For intentional delay or stalling, PENALTY: 5-Off.

15. A cue slipping from a player's hand which touches any live disc PENALTY: 10-Off plus any 10-Offs the offender has on the board. Other good discs of the offender shall not count. Opponent's good discs on the court, prior to the offense, shall be credited to the opponent's score, except any 10-Offs and the half-round shall be played over unless game point has been reached by opponent.

15a. A cue which slips from a player's hand and which ends up on another court, interfering with player shooting a disc on that court, or which moves or touches a live disc on a court other than the offender's court, PENALTY: 10-Off to offender losing control of cue and round shall be played over on the court where the offense took place with no score being credited to any player. If no live discs have been disturbed the player interfered with may take their shot over. (Approved Mar 2004, reworded for clarity 2007).

15b. A dead disc coming from another court which interferes with a disc being shot from a court other than the offender's court: PENATLY 10-Off to offender. If a live disc shot, other than the disc shot, is touched by the errant disc the half-round on the court where the disc was touched shall be played over with no score being credited to any player. If the only disc touched by the errant disc is the one being shot by the player on the other court, the player shooting may take his shot over and the half-round shall not be played over.

16. NO HESITATION SHOT ALLOWED. PENATLY: 10-Off. Any 10-Off(s) the offender had on the court were displaced will be removed before further play and also be deducted from offender's score.

17. NO HOOK SHOT ALLOWED. The shot must be delivered in a straight line with continuous forward motion of the cue and disc. PENATLY: 10-Off, offender's disc removed, and opponent credited with score of any of his/her discs displaced. All displaced discs shall be removed from the court immediately after scorings of opponent's displaced discs. Any 10-Off the offender had on the court that was displaced will be removed before further play and also be deducted from offender's score.

17a. Regarding a hook shot, hesitation shot, shooting off from line, there will be no appeal, as there is only one person who can tell if you have shot off the line or made a hook or hesitation shot, and that is the referee. That is strictly a judgment call by the referee, and once he/she has made that call, it will stand. The only time a divisional should be called is if the referee isn't sure of the penalty or gives wrong penalty – then the player will make an appeal.

18. Any player shooting two consecutive discs, PENALTY: 10-Off, plus any 10-Offs offender may have on court. Other good discs of offender will not count. Opponent credited with all good discs on court before second disc played (except 10-Off) and that half-round played over unless game point has been reached by offender's opponent.

.

19. In case of improper action of a player not specifically covered by the rules, or in a match to which court referee has not been assigned, the Tournament Director will ascertain the facts and may assess a penalty. He/She will also insure that the offender gains no advantage from his/her improper action and, in addition, impose a 10-Off Penalty.

20. A disc or discs returning or remaining on the playing area of the court, after having struck any object outside the playing area, shall be removed before further play. It is called a dead disc.

20a. If a dead disc rebounds or ricochets and touches a live disc, or causes another dead disc to touch a live disc, the half-round shall be played over and a 10-Off PENALTY to the player shooting the offending disc causing the replay. [Rest of rule deleted – Approved by FSA Board 10-14-2006].

20b. If a dead disc coming from another court moves or displaces a live disc, that half-round shall be played over, with no score credited to any player. A 10-Off PENALTY to the player on another court shooting the offending disc causing the half-round to be played over.

20c. Player shooting a disc making one or more discs to go completely over the backstop or rebounding from over the backstop, PENALTY: 10-Off. This rule is temporarily suspended. The Florida Shuffleboard Association MAY, by a majority vote of the entire Executive Board, reinstate the 20c Hard Shooting Rule AT ANY TIME.

21. Any disc that clearly leaves the court beyond the farthest baseline, or goes off the sides of the court is a dead disc.

22. A disc, which stops less than eight inches (8") beyond the farthest baseline, shall be removed.

23. A disc that is leaning over the edge of court and touching the alley shall be immediately removed.

24. A match will be forfeited after the third call of 5-minute intervals, total 15 minutes, starting from the time that a playable court is available.

25. Any team or individual that forfeits or is forfeited in a game or match, up to and including the quarter-finals, is DISQUALIFIED from the tournament.

26. No electronic equipment (cell phones, etc) allowed on court - PENALTY of 5-points assessed for unauthorized use.

D – Scoring

1. SCORING DIAGRAM – one 10-point area; two 8-point areas; two 7-point areas; one 10-Off area.

2. After both players have shot their four (4) discs, SCORE ALL discs on diagram within and NOT touching lines; separation triangle in 10-Off area not considered.

JUDGING DISC: When judging disc in relation to lines, the official shall position himself/herself with the disc between him/her and the line and sight DIRECTLY DOWN.

A MOUNTED DISC, or resting on top of disc, happens sometimes when players use excessive force in shooting. Each disc shall be judged separately according to scoring rules.

No Artificial Aid or Cue shall be used in judging discs. Use EYESIGHT ONLY, except in judging lagging discs. PENALTY: 5-Off.

3. Play continues until all discs have been shot in that half-round, even if game has been reached.

4. If a tie game results at game point or over, play is continued in regular rotation of play, until two full rounds in doubles or one full round in singles are completed. At that time the side with the higher score wins, even if it has less than 75 points or the number of points specified as game points.

5. In tournament play, the winner of a match must sign the score card, thus approving the record entered thereon.

6. If an error occurs in the scoring of a score on the scoreboard at the end of a half-round and it is discovered before the next half-round is completed, the error must be corrected. Otherwise the score as scored on the scoreboard must stand, unless both sides are agreed on the correction.

E - Officials

1. Officials in Tournament Play shall be Tournament Director, Assistant to the Tournament Director, Divisional Referees, Court Referees and Court Scorers.

1a. A Court Referee shall be assigned to a match upon the request of any player in that match.

2. THE TOURNAMENT DIRECTOR shall have complete charge of arrangements of the tournament-namely, conduct the drawings, pairings, assign the courts, officials, set time for starting games and matches; inspect all courts and equipment, etc., and all other details which enter into tournament play. The Tournament Director may also cancel, suspend, or otherwise re-arrange court calls and tournament play in such instances where extreme weather conditions prevail.

3. An ASSISTANT to the TOURNAMENT DIRECTOR may be appointed as desired by the Tournament Director. He/She shall render final call on close discs (third call), shall render decisions on question of fact, but final APPEAL FROM PLAYERS will be made by the Tournament director.

4. DIVISIONAL REFEREE: One or more Divisional Referees shall be appointed, number dependent on how many courts are in play.

    The Divisional Referees are the aides of the Tournament Director, and shall carry out his/her orders regarding assigning officials and players to courts. He/She shall see that discs, indicators, pointers, chalk, score cards, and other necessary equipment are at each court. He/She shall inform officials of any special rules and regulations which have been made for the conducting of the tournament. He/She shall collect all score cards at finish of matches and shall return them to the Tournament Director. He/She shall have jurisdiction only on the action of courts assigned to him/her. Divisional referees shall be informed by Court Referees of all PLAYER APPEALS and, if decision made by Court Referee is not justified or not according to the rules, may over-rule him/her.

    If a Divisional Referee observes a violation of a rule by a player in his/her assigned section in a match on a court without and assigned Referee, the Divisional Referee will notify the Tournament Director of the violation. With the Tournament Director's approval, the Divisional Referee will assign a Referee to that court for the remainder of the match.

5. COURT REFEREE shall have complete charge of play on court assigned to him/her. He/She shall consult his/her Divisional Referee on APPEALS FROM PLAYERS. He/She shall be sole authority on decisions and scores, except as above noted. He/She shall inform players of any rules and regulations made for the tournament. He/She shall give signal for start of play, shall call disc good or no count, shall remove dead discs from play, shall announce score at end of each play, shall have charge of color indicator and announce color lead. He/She shall announce any violation of rules to players and instruct scorer as to penalty of same. He/She shall supervise the scoring and assure himself/herself that it is correctly done.

HE/she shall not touch live discs in determining whether they are good or no count. If He/She should disturb live discs, half-round played over. He/She shall not gather discs for the players, He/She shall sign score card at end of match and verify that scores are correct.

For any rule violation seen by the Referee, a fine must be mandatory, with Referee giving no warning at any time in all tournaments.

6. COURT SCORER shall tally clearly the score of game on scoreboard at end of court, tallying only score called by Court Referee after each half-round.

F - Appeals

1. Either player in singles, and either player in doubles at the end of the court to which the discs are played, may:

    Request permission from the Referee to examine any close disc as to good or not good, or;

    Ask the Referee if a disc is close and the Referee responds "Yes"; this automatic approval for the player to examine it without additional approval. In singles, when there is no referee on the court, a player may go and examine the disc as to good or not good, and also to gain information concerning location of discs.

1a. If a player wishes to make an appeal on any close disc, as to whether it is good or no count, it must be made before another disc is shot by either player, and the decision made shall be final and cannot be again appealed at the end of the half-round, unless such disc or discs have been touched or moved by another disc after decision was made. Anyone from the shooting end of the court in doubles asking for either First or Second Call shall be construed as coaching. PENALTY: 10-Off.

1b. If the Referee and Divisional agree, there will be no third call. If they disagree, there must be a third call by the Director or his/her representative.

1c. If there has been no request by either party to examine a close disc until AFTER the half-round is completed, then the half-round is played over if either player protests the Referee's call, and the protest is sustained by the Tournament Director, UNLESS such disc or discs protested is (are) the result of the last disc played. No live disc will be moved after a disc has been protested and no dead disc may be placed in the playing area, until the protested disc has been finalized. PENALTY: 10-Off.

1d. Shooter may ask Referee to have partner check close disc. If there is no Referee, shooter may ask partner to check the close disc.

2. Player or players making appeal without sufficient reason shall be PENALIZED 10 POINTS OFF SCORE.

3. Players may request officials to give them information concerning location of discs. Players shall not be permitted to examine these discs.

4. A player or team may protest any one or more officials assigned to their court, provided such protest is placed before the Divisional Referee or Tournament Director before the first game begins.

5.   To refuse assignment of a Referee, a player or team must have a good and valid stated reason.

      Note: Tournament Director or Divisional Referee must appoint other officials to serve in place of those protested, which appointment must stand.

G – Substitutes

1.   Once a tournament starts, there will be no substitutes allowed in any tournament in the State of Florida. Tournament starts when the draw is complete.

H – Wet Courts

1.   If it starts to rain during any unfinished half-round of play, players will not be required to complete the half-round. All discs will be removed from court to a dry place. In case of rain, Scorekeeper will write on the back of the scorecard the scores, color lead, and at which end of the court play will resume. If the Tournament Director decides that the game is to continue after the rain ceases, play will then be resumed at score and color lead where play ceased. (If half-round was not completed, then half-round will be played over).

2.   If Tournament Director shall deem it necessary to discontinue play on account of weather conditions, any unfinished game or match shall be resumed later, at score and color lead where play ceased.

3.   Practice after a rain delay is to be as follows: If play can restart on the same day, there will be two (2) speed shots and four (4) practice discs. If play restarts the following day, there will be full practice including two (2) speed shots.

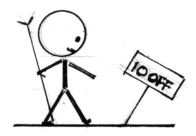

I – Violations and Penalties

C-3b	Shooting opponent's disc	10-Off	
C-4a	Discs not in starting area	5-Off	
C-4b	Played disc touching front or back line	5-Off	
C-4c	Played disc touching sides of triangle	10-Off	(see Rule 4c)
C-5	Players stepping on or over baseline or extension of baseline while in the act of shooting	10-Off	
C-5a	Player must not touch any part of body on or over baseline at any time while executing a shot	10-Off	
C-6	Players must not stand or step on adjoining court	5-Off	
C-7	Players not remaining seated	5-Off	
C-8	Players must not leave court during game without permission except to gather discs	10-Off	
C-9	Standing in way or equipment in way of opponent	5-Off	
C-9a	Fail to step to the rear with cue in vertical position	5-Off	
C-10	Touching live disc (see Rule 10 for total PENALTY)	10-Off	(see Rule 10)
C-11	Remarks disconcerting opponent	10-Off	
C-12	Any remark or motion to partner	10-Off	
C-13	Shooting disc while opponent's disc in motion	10-Off	(see Rule 13)
C-14	For intentional stalling	5-Off	
C-15	Cue slipping from player's hand	10-Off	(see Rule 15/15a/15b)
C-16	No hesitation shot allowed	10-Off	(see Rule 16/17a)
C-17	No hook shot allowed	10-Off	(see Rule 17/17a)
C-18	Player shooting two consecutive discs	10-Off	(see Rule 18)
C-19	For improper action, not otherwise covered, Tournament Director may impose Penalty which prevents any advantage to violator, plus Penalty	10-Off	
C-20a	Player shooting disc rebounds causing replay of half-round	10-Off	
C-20b	Player shooting disc rebounds causing replay of another court	10-Off	
C-20c	Disc going over backstop is TEMPORARILY SUSPENDED		
C-25	Forfeit before semifinal DISQUALIFIED		
C-26	Unauthorized electronic equipment	5-Off	
D-2	No artificial aid/cue when judging disc	5-Off	
F-1a	Shooting ends in doubles asking for a call. Considered Coaching	10-Off	
F-1c	Moving disputed disc before inspection	10-Off	
F-2	Appealing without reason	10-Off	

SHUFFLEBOARD COURT MAINTENANCE:

Court Maintenance:

The enjoyment and success of playing Shuffleboard depends upon the condition of the court surface. The ideal playing surface, the discs SLIDE fast/true and require a minimum amount of force to propel the disc towards the opposite end of the court, to score/prevent the opponent from scoring or both.

Courts which are slow, spotty or too fast cause over shooting which results in shooting yourself into the kitchen or the lack of speed to reach the intended target. Also, leaves the opponent's disc on the court or overshoot the intended target.

Slow courts cause fatigue/difficult to execute carom or combination shots. Courts which have an over dose of glass beads are extremely fast which causes erratic trajectory of the discs and hard to judge the speed.

The ideal concrete court is level with a sand or carpet finish surface, patio green color with sharp white lines marking the court layout. On regular basis the court maintenance as recommended by Allen R. Shuffleboard Inc., 6595 Seminole Blvd., Seminole, FL 33772 1-800-260-3834 Mrshuffle1@aol.com as follows:

1. Sweep the courts daily.
2. Hose the courts weekly with clean water.
3. Twice a year, wash the courts with a good liquid soap.
4. Wax the courts two (2) to three (3) times a year with Nella-#2 Court Wax. Use a 12" lambs wool applicator or paint roller. Most clubs apply 2-coats. One (1) gallon of Nella-Seal- #2 Court wax will cover two (2) coats per court.

Other Products which are available to improve playing conditions are:
1. Krystal Glaze – Acrylic shuffleboard base coating. A water-based crystal clear product for sealing a court. 1-gallon will cover four (4) courts. Apply product after line painting is completed.
2. Shuffle Glass Beads – Popular court dressing. Sprinkle sparingly on the court. Sold in 6 lb and 12 lb containers.
3. Disc Wax – Excellent disc conditioner. Apply 6-lines Horizontally and 6-lines vertically (checkerboard fashion) to the bottom of the Shuffleboard discs. Also to the outer rim of the bottom of the discs.
4. Plastic- Beads- - Manufactured by Dura-Dress Co., CA, known as "California Slush." Sold in 5 lb units. Sprinkle sparingly on the court. (#4035-W/R 30).

To build Concrete Shuffleboard Courts in Florida contact the following:
Nidy Built Courts
P.O. Box 730
Sanford, FL 32772
1-800-226-6439
www.shuffleboardsupplies.com

CLOSING THOUGHTS

Suggestions which may help to make your shuffleboard game more enjoyable and productive in winning games.

1. Select a point and aim for this point when trying to block or guard a disc. A rule of thumb, try to keep about 5 to 6 feet between the stationary disc and your point of aim.
2. You have the hammer: be conservative, score for points. Often a score of 7 or 8 will add up for a win.
3. Before shooting: look for a hide behind your opponent's disc.
4. Keep the board <u>CLEAN</u> when playing against a <u>Kitchen Player</u>.
5. Protect a leading score with a block or a guard disc.
6. Waste the hammer when not needed for a score.
7. Waste the # 6 disc when you are ahead in the score and the board is clean.
8. Seldom try to kitchen a St. Pete.
9. Watch for the drift when trying a kitchen shot in the low 7-area.
10. When to use a combination shot versus a carom shot: Remember at 45 degrees these shots are similar.

Remember: The classic game of Shuffleboard: clean the board, scoring the hammer will win more games the majority of times.

Lady Luck: Luck always plays a part in all games!! Luck goes both ways, for and against you. Generally the player who makes the better shots and uses the best strategy wins.

Remember: Shuffleboard is the only game in which you can reduce your opponent's score and at the same time increase your score. **ALWAYS! ALWAYS! ALWAYS!** <u>LOOK</u> at the **SCORE BOARD** before you **SHOOT**.

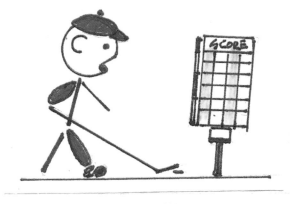

MY FRIEND !!!

GLOSSARY

GLOSSARY of TERMS

Alley _____ The entire length of the court, between the St. Pete and the edge of the court.

Apex _____ The apex of the triangle,10-area.

Backstop _____ A disc that is placed that can serve to stop a cue disc for a score.

Bait _____ Place a disc in the scoring area, kitchen bait .

Baseline _____ The line which separates the minus 10 line from the player's standing line.

Beads _____ Fine sand/plastic beads sprinkled on a court to reduce the friction between the court surface and the moving discs.

BLACK Court _____ The direction of the drift favors BLACK .

Blast _____ Shooting very hard, generally in tournaments to avoid sticking.

Block _____ A disc used to protect a scored disc.

Blocking Game _____ Placing a Tampa block after a St. Pete has been placed by the opponent, in lieu of clearing the board.

Board _____ The court area between the lag line and the base line.

Bump Shot _____ Hitting a disc not on the scoring field into a scoring position.

Bunny _____ A disc which is the winning score.

Carom _____ The cue disc strikes the target disc, and moves on a different course to another target.

Clear the Board _____ Shot which removes both discs from the court.

Close Disc _____ A disc so close to the line it is difficult to determine whether it scores.

Color Lead _____ The color, YELLOW/BLACK, of the first disc to be played in a frame.

Combination _____ A cue disc strikes a second disc to move it to strike a third disc.

Court Officials _____ Tournament manager/court referee/court umpire and court scorer.

Cross Guard _____ Cross Guard the same as a St. Pete.

Court _____ The playing area (see court diagram).

Cue Stick _____ Stick to shoot a disc.

Dead Disc _____ A disc that leaves the court or fails to reach the dead line is dead. If the disc *stops* on, or just touches it is a *live* disc. A disc over the edge of the court is *not dead* until it falls of its own weight into the the gutter. A dead disc lying on the court, or against the court, must be removed before the next play.

Dead Line _____ A line three (3) feet in front of the apex of the 10-area triangle.

Deep _____ See High/Low.

Delivery _____ The act of shooting a disc.

Disc _____ Discs used in the game of shuffleboard, 4-YELLOW/4-BLACK, 8 make a set.

Double _____ A shot which scores both the cue disc and the liner of the same color.

Drift _____ Disc deviates from a straight line due to the slant of the court which may not be visible to the eye.

End Game _____ Last part of game with hammer and without hammer.

Fast Shot _____ Shot with speed to clear the board.

Fast Court _____ Very fast court, the discs move freely without too much effort.

Foot _____ End of the court, opposite the scoreboard.

Foul Line _____ The back line of the minus 10 area.

Frame _____ Frame, shuffleboard game, that starts at the Head of the court, each player shoots four (4) discs.

Fun Game _____ Same meaning as Friendly Game, this is not a tournament, some win some lose!

Game Point _____ Scored disc making the total score 75; or any number of points determined by the players.

Glance _____ A shot by the cue disc, has impact with the target, changes course and stops in a favorable spot for a score.

Good Shot _____ Any shot that does what is intended.

Guard _____ A disc is placed to create protection for the next shot. Or a disc is placed to stop the play by the opponent.

Hammer _____ Disc # 8; the last disc in the round of play.

Handle _____ A second disc beyond a guard which protrudes enough to be hit by your opponent's disc to spoil both scores with a combination shot.

Head _____ The score board at the end of the court.

Hide _____ A disc placed behind another disc which can serve as protection against a straight shot.

High/Low _____ High/Low refers to the position of the disc in the scoring area. High 10/ High 8/ High 7 refer to a disc that stops just over the line, leaving a space too small for the opponent to score while knocking away the disc. Deep 10/8/7 and deep (-10) refer to discs that are near the far side of these areas, allowing room for the opponent to score by using the discs as backstops.

GLOSSARY of TERMS

Hook Shot — A cue shot changes direction during delivery.

Kitchen — The 10-Off area of the scoring area.

Kitchen Bait — A disc placed deep in the 7-area, without protection, to get the opponent to shoot at the disc and put it into the kitchen.

Kitchen Player — Player who tries at every opportunity to move the opponent's disc into the 10-Off area.

Kitchen Speed — The speed required to put the opponent's disc into the kitchen.

Kitchen-speed(+) — Speed of a cue disc faster than kitchen speed to carry opponent's disc off the scoring area for sure and into the kitchen if the shooter should error on the slow side.

Kiss Shot — Touch a disc on a line into a score area.

Lag — To shoot for choice of color before a tournament game begins.

Liner — A live disc lying on a line.

Lose the Hammer — Player with hammer fails to score during their round of play.

Magic Circle — The scoring level of two (2) numbers (about 15 points) from game point. Game of 75, 60 is considered to be the lower limit of the magic circle.

Maintenance — yearly and daily care of the shuffleboard playing surface. See Chapter 17.

Match Play — In a tournament, one (1) player wins, one(1) player goes home. In league play, a complete number of games is played by team A versus team B.

Modular System — The system, the brackets, "climb the stairs."

Module — A range of scores used in the system, bracket.

Nick — The cue disc unintentional striking another disc on the board.

Out — Who shoots first? BLACK is out means BLACK shoots first.

Pigeon — A disc on the 7 and 10-Off line, a sitting duck.

Playing the Drift — Compensating for the drift to make a shot the same as one which would have been made on a level court.

Play Dumb — Fail to use good sense, fail to do what is proper.

Point Game — A game with a predetermined score to win.

Round — In **doubles** or walking **singles**, a round is 16 frames, 8 from the Head, 8 from the Foot. In non-walking singles, a round of 16 frames, all on the same end of the court, either the Head/or Foot. A half round of a game in doubles/or singles in which 8 frames are played from either end of the court.

Rush the Game — Take unnecessary risk near the end of the game by trying to get an extra score on the board to bring the game to a premature close.

St. Pete — A disc placed in front of the opponent's side of the scoring triangle.

Separation Line — All lines which divide the playing field into scoring areas.

Separate triangle — In the center of the 10-Off area a wedge-shaped lines which separates the yellow and black discs at the beginning of each half frame.

Shot — To propel a disc with a cue-stick.

Sighting — Take aim at the target before shooting.

Sneak — A disc shot into the scoring area behind a St. Pete or Tampa or a block for a hide.

Snuggle — Place a scoring disc close behind one of the opponent's disc for protection.

Steal a Hammer — when a player scores in a frame, the opponent has the hammer and fails to score.

Stick — To stop on the board (cue disc) in almost the same spot as the disc which was knocked away.

Suicide Alley — The entire length of the court lying between the St. Pete and the outer edge of the court.

Table — The playing court scoring area, see (Board).

Tampa — A guard placed close to the apex on the shooter's side of the court.

Target — The disc at which the cue disc is aimed.

Up – Down Shot — The player's disc hits the opponent's good 10, sticks for a good 10 and puts the other disc in the kitchen for a minus 10.

YELLOW Court — A court on which the moving discs drift towards the BLACK side of the court. The direction of the drift favors the player of the YELLOW discs.

INDEX

INDEX

CPSIA information can be obtained
at www.ICGtesting.com
Printed in the USA
LVIW021338260313
326099LV00005BB

* 9 7 8 1 5 8 9 0 9 9 0 8 1 *